Intensive
Diabetes Management

FIFTH EDITION

Edited by
Joseph I. Wolfsdorf, MB BCh

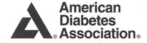
**American
Diabetes
Association.**

Director, Book Publishing, Abe Ogden; *Managing Editor*, Greg Guthrie; *Acquisitions Editor*, Victor Van Beuren; *Editor*, Rebekah Renshaw; *Production Manager*, Melissa Sprott; *Composition*, ADA; *Cover Design*, Jody Billert; *Printer*, Versa Press.

Printed in the United States of America
1 3 5 7 9 10 8 6 4 2

The suggestions and information contained in this publication are generally consistent with the *Clinical Practice Recommendations* and other policies of the American Diabetes Association, but they do not represent the policy or position of the Association or any of its boards or committees. Reasonable steps have been taken to ensure the accuracy of the information presented. However, the American Diabetes Association cannot ensure the safety or efficacy of any product or service described in this publication. Individuals are advised to consult a physician or other appropriate health care professional before undertaking any diet or exercise program or taking any medication referred to in this publication. Professionals must use and apply their own professional judgment, experience, and training and should not rely solely on the information contained in this publication before prescribing any diet, exercise, or medication. The American Diabetes Association—its officers, directors, employees, volunteers, and members—assumes no responsibility or liability for personal or other injury, loss, or damage that may result from the suggestions or information in this publication.

♾ The paper in this publication meets the requirements of the ANSI Standard Z39.48-1992 (permanence of paper).

ADA titles may be purchased for business or promotional use or for special sales. To purchase more than 50 copies of this book at a discount, or for custom editions of this book with your logo, contact the American Diabetes Association at the address below, at booksales@diabetes.org, or by calling 703-299-2046.

American Diabetes Association
1701 North Beauregard Street
Alexandria, Virginia 22311

DOI: 10.2337/9781580404587

Library of Congress Cataloging-in-Publication Data
Intensive diabetes management / Joseph I. Wolfsdorf, editor. -- 5th ed.
    p. ; cm.
  Includes bibliographical references and index.
  Summary: "This is the most current and practical book available on how to begin and maintain intensive diabetes management"--Provided by publisher.
  ISBN 978-1-58040-458-7 (pbk. : alk. paper)
  I. Wolfsdorf, Joseph I.. II. American Diabetes Association.
  [DNLM: 1. Diabetes Mellitus--therapy. 2. Diabetic Diet. 3. Insulin--administration & dosage. 4. Patient Education as Topic. 5. Self Care--methods. WK 815]
  616.4'62--dc23
                                                                2012009317

Contents

Monitoring   137

Nutrition Management   149

A Word About This Guide

This fifth edition of *Intensive Diabetes Management* is one of the many books for clinicians published by the American Diabetes Association. Other titles include *Medical Management of Type 1 Diabetes*, *Medical Management of Type 2 Diabetes*, *Therapy for Diabetes Mellitus and Related Disorders*, and *Managing Preexisting Diabetes and Pregnancy*. These books provide health care professionals with the comprehensive information needed to give the best possible medical care to patients with diabetes.

Intensive Diabetes Management focuses on the intensive management of patients with type 1 or type 2 diabetes. The idea for this book was first conceived during discussions with colleagues regarding implementation of the results of the Diabetes Control and Complications Trial (DCCT). The goal was to present a practical guide for clinical care and patient education, with emphasis on the team approach to diabetes care and comprehensive self-management education.

The 19 years since the publication of the DCCT results have seen enormous changes in professional and lay approaches to diabetes management. Striving for more intensive management is now commonplace rather than the exception in diabetes care, and management approaches considered "experimental" in the DCCT are now standards of care in clinical diabetes practice. This book will provide all diabetes care professionals the tools to provide each patient with as intensive a diabetes management plan as each patient is ready and able to incorporate into his or her diabetes management strategy.

Most patients with diabetes will benefit from care by professionals knowledgeable in the principles of intensive diabetes management, even those patients not yet ready for the full "package" of intensive management. It is the hope of those who contributed to the current edition that healthcare professionals who care for patients with diabetes will recognize "teachable moments" and strive to intensify their patients' diabetes management with treatment goals appropriate for each patient's skills and medical condition.

All contributors are experts in their respective fields and are daily involved in helping patients intensify their diabetes management. They offer the approaches to intensive diabetes management that they have found to be of most benefit to patients. They share their techniques and strategies for success, including altering treatment regimens and glycemic goals to the patient's needs and abilities. This is the most current and practical book available on how to begin and maintain intensive diabetes management. The contributors have based their recommendations on the results of the DCCT, subsequent studies of individual aspects of intensive diabetes management, the United Kingdom Prospective Diabetes Study, and the American Diabetes Association's Clinical Practice Recommendations.

We hope that this updated edition of *Intensive Diabetes Management* will be as useful an addition to your professional library as the previous editions and that it will inspire you to incorporate the knowledge and skills presented here into your clinical practice. All health professionals who care for people with diabetes will find guidance for implementing the improved diabetes care we know is so valuable.

Finally, I wish to dedicate the fifth edition to the numerous diabetes nurse educators, dietitians, mental health professionals, and physician colleagues.

JOSEPH I. WOLFSDORF, MB, BCH
Editor

Contributors to the Fifth Edition

Roberta Capelson, ANP
Manager of Diabetes Outreach
Boston Medical Center
Clinical Instructor
Boston University School of Medicine

Gayle M. Lorenzi, RN, CDE
Community Health Project Manager
University of California, San Diego

James L. Rosenzweig, MD
Director of Diabetes Services
Boston Medical Center
Associate Professor of Medicine
Boston University School of Medicine

Barbara Schreiner, PhD, RN,
  CDE, BC-ADM

Suzanne Strowig, MSN, RN, CDE
Diabetes Clinical Nurse Specialist
Faculty Associate
University of Texas Southwestern Medical
  Center
Department of Internal Medicine

Joseph I. Wolfsdorf, MB, BCh
Clinical Director and Associate Chief,
Director, Diabetes Program
Division of Endocrinology, Children's
Hospital Boston
Professor of Pediatrics, Harvard Medical
  School

Howard Wolpert, MB, BCh
Senior Physician, Section of Adult Diabetes
Director, Insulin Pump & CGM Programs
Joslin Diabetes Center
Assistant Professor of Medicine
Harvard Medical School

Deborah Young-Hyman, Ph.D.
Professor of Pediatrics
Georgia Prevention Institute
Georgia Health Sciences University

Acknowledgments

The American Diabetes Association gratefully acknowledges the contributions of the following health care professionals and members of the Association's Professional Section to previous editions of this work:

Ruth Farkas-Hirsch, MS, RN, CDE (editor, 2nd edition); Betty Page Brackenridge, MS, RD, CDE; and Neil H. White, MD, CDE; as well as Georgeanna J. Klingensmith, MD (editor, 3rd edition); Karen M. Bolderman, RD, LD, CDE; Rodney A. Lorenz, MD; Gail Spiegel, MS, RD, CDE; Fred W. Whitehouse, MD, MACP; and Philip Zeitler, MD, PhD.

Terminology of Intensive Diabetes Management

- **Type 1 diabetes:** a disorder that results from a progressive destruction of the pancreatic β-cells (insulitis) and leads to a permanent insulin-dependent state; usually the result of an autoimmune disorder

- **Type 2 diabetes:** a nonautoimmune disorder caused by a combination of peripheral insulin resistance and varying degrees of insulin deficiency in which ~50% of patients ultimately require insulin; most likely has multiple causes

- **Gestational diabetes:** a form of glucose intolerance first identified during pregnancy

- **Intensive diabetes management:** a mode of treatment for the person with diabetes that has the goal of achieving euglycemia or near-normal glycemia, using all available resources to accomplish this goal

- **Glycemic goal:** glycated hemoglobin (A1C) <7.0% and blood glucose levels that fall within the range of 90–130 mg/dl (5.0–7.2 mmol/l) preprandially and not exceeding <180 mg/dl (<10 mmol/l) postprandially

- **Euglycemia:** blood glucose levels that fall within the nondiabetic range

- **Improved glycemic control:** lower levels of A1C and mean blood glucose than during a previous course of diabetes therapy

- **Diabetes team:** health care professionals from different disciplines who actively work with a patient with diabetes to achieve common goals of management; the team generally includes a physician, nurse manager/educator/clinician, dietitian, mental health professional, and other specialists as needed, all experienced in the care of people with diabetes

- **Basal insulin:** an intermediate-acting (NPH) or long-acting (glargine or detemir) insulin that is more slowly absorbed from a subcutaneous depot into the bloodstream, mimicking secretion of insulin by pancreatic β-cells in the postabsorptive period; or the background insulin (regular, lispro, glulisine, or aspart) given continuously by an insulin pump

- **Bolus insulin:** regular insulin or a rapid-acting insulin analog (lispro, glulisine, or aspart) injected at the time of food intake to permit a rapid rise in free plasma insulin level after a meal, mimicking the postprandial secretion of insulin by pancreatic β-cells and blunting the rise in blood glucose; or the prandial insulin dose delivered by an insulin pump

■ **Insulin infusion pump:** a continuous subcutaneous insulin infusion (CSII) system that delivers rapid-acting insulin in an open-loop fashion into a subcutaneous site from a computer-driven, externally mounted reservoir

■ **Multiple doses of insulin (MDI):** a management strategy for insulin delivery that includes the use of three or more injections of insulin daily to provide both basal and bolus insulin requirements

■ **Lag time:** that period (in minutes) between the subcutaneous injection of regular or rapid-acting insulin and its initially effective physiological action, which varies both by insulin and from person to person as well as in the same person from time to time

■ **Open-loop insulin delivery:** a system of insulin delivery that is independent of the moment-to-moment changes in plasma glucose levels, the only type available to the patient with diabetes in 2012

■ **Closed-loop insulin delivery:** a system of insulin delivery wherein insulin is released into the bloodstream in response to the moment-to-moment change in the plasma glucose level, i.e., pancreatic β-cell insulin delivery

■ **Implantable intraperitoneal insulin delivery system:** a means of open-loop insulin delivery from a subcutaneously implanted, computer-driven insulin reservoir surgically placed in the abdominal wall with a delivery line threaded into the peritoneal cavity

■ **Hypoglycemia unawareness:** the inability of a person with diabetes to know when blood glucose has declined to a hazardously low level

■ **Carbohydrate counting:** a method of tracking nutritional intake of carbohydrates and relating the carbohydrate quantity to an insulin dosage, e.g., 1 unit rapid-acting insulin is needed for each 5–25 g carbohydrate consumed; key aspect of intensive management that requires education of and personalization for the patient

■ **Continuous subcutaneous glucose monitoring system:** a minimally invasive technique that frequently measures interstitial tissue glucose levels, permitting analysis of glucose variation over several days

Rationale for and Physiological Basis of Intensive Diabetes Management

---

Highlights
Rationale for and Physiological Basis of Intensive Diabetes Management

- Technological and pharmacological innovations have made it possible for individuals with diabetes to achieve near-normal glycemic control.

- The goal of intensive diabetes management is to achieve near-normal glycemia. This mode of treatment has been shown in large prospective randomized studies as the preferred approach for many patients with diabetes to delay the onset of microalbuminuria and the progression of micro- to macroalbuminuria in patients with both type 1 and type 2 diabetes.

- Glycemic control that approaches the nondiabetic state postpones or slows the progression of the retinal, renal, neurological, and macrovascular complications of diabetes.

- Glycemic control that approaches that of the nondiabetic state lowers risk factors that promote macrovascular disease (e.g., plasminogen activator inhibitor–1 levels; platelet aggregation; small, dense low-density lipoprotein [LDL] cholesterol particles).

- Intensive diabetes management is successful when insulin is delivered and adjusted in amounts required by changes in nutritional intake (e.g., amounts of carbohydrate, protein, fat), physical activity, and associated internal and external stresses. Successful management of these issues will approximate normal fuel metabolism.

- Self monitoring of blood glucose is performed to guide adjustments in insulin dosage in relation to food consumption and, especially, carbohydrate intake, activity variation, and ambient blood glucose level to achieve the following:
  - a relatively constant, low plasma free insulin level during fasting (postabsorptive state)
  - a rapid increase in plasma free insulin after meals, in an amount appropriate to the amount of food (primarily carbohydrate) eaten
  - a decrease in plasma free insulin levels especially during and after prolonged, strenuous exercise or when food intake is delayed

Rationale for and Physiological Basis of Intensive Diabetes Management

Diabetes management aims to achieve near-normal glycemic control to prevent or ameliorate diabetes complications. The effectiveness of glycemic control in reducing the risk of microvascular and neuropathic complications is well established. Technical advances such as self-monitoring of blood glucose (SMBG), the measurement of glycated hemoglobin (A1c), continuous glucose monitoring (CGM), insulin analogs, and the availability of technically advanced "smart" insulin pumps have provided the tools for successful intensive diabetes management.

Studies in type 1 diabetes, type 2 diabetes, and in pregnant women with diabetes have shown benefits sufficient to prompt a consensus on intensive glycemic control as a standard of care. The landmark Diabetes Control and Complications Trial (DCCT) showed that glycemic control (achieving mean A1c of 7.1%) postpones, prevents, or slows the progression of retinal, renal, and neurological complications. Follow-up of the DCCT cohort in the Epidemiology of Diabetes Interventions and Complications (EDIC) study has shown persistence of the beneficial effects in the intensively treated subjects even though their glycemic control during follow-up has been equivalent to that of subjects in the conventional treatment arm of the DCCT. Glucose lowering in the intensive treatment arm was also associated with long-term benefit with regard to cardiovascular complications. Intensive treatment, therefore, should be started as soon as is safely possible after the onset of type 1 diabetes and maintained thereafter aiming for a practicable target A1c level of 7.0% or less provided that this can be achieved safely and without frequent and severe hypoglycemia.

In type 2 diabetes, the United Kingdom Prospective Diabetes Study (UKPDS) in patients with new-onset type 2 diabetes and the Kumamoto Study in Japan, similarly, demonstrated significant reductions in microvascular and neuropathic complications with intensive therapy. The majority of patients with diabetes succumb to heart attack, stroke, or their consequences. The potential of intensive glycemic control to reduce cardiovascular disease in type 2 diabetes is supported by epidemiological studies and a meta-analysis. Three randomized controlled trials (the Action to Control Cardiovascular Risk in Diabetes [ACCORD], Action in Diabetes and Vascular Disease: Preterax and Diamicron Modified Release Controlled Evaluation [ADVANCE], and Veterans Affairs Diabetes Trial [VADT]), however, showed that targeting near-normal A1c in high-risk patients with type 2 diabetes did not have a beneficial effect on cardiovascular disease. Indeed, a treatment strategy designed to lower blood glucose to near-normal levels in the ACCORD trial was associated with increased mortality.

3

Table 1.1 Benefits of Successful Intensive Diabetes Management

- More predictable blood glucose values
- Lowered risk of microvascular complications developing and/or progressing
- Improved plasma lipid levels and leukocyte function
- Lowered maternal and fetal morbidity and/or mortality during pregnancy
- Diminished risk of congenital malformations in the fetus
- Optimal linear growth and physical development in children
- Better control of the dawn phenomenon
- A feeling of physical and emotional well-being and of "being in control"
- Greater freedom of lifestyle and daily schedule
- Greater knowledge and insight into diabetes care

Although glucose management clearly is important, aggressive management of blood pressure and lipids, smoking cessation, and antiplatelet therapy are also critically important aspects of care, can dramatically reduce the rate of cardiovascular events, and must also be a major focus of therapy.

Table 1.1 shows benefits of intensive diabetes management; Table 1.2 summarizes some of the adverse effects of this approach. Severe hypoglycemia and weight gain are the leading potential adverse effects of intensified glycemic control. The increased frequency of hypoglycemia begins at initiation of intensive management and persists as long as it is continued.

Intensive management strategies have been increasingly adopted by patients with type 1 diabetes across the age spectrum as well as in many patients with type 2 diabetes. Indeed, some elderly patients with longstanding type 2 diabetes experience control resembling that of an insulin deficient patient, having wide swings of blood glucose, and sensitivity to timing or small differences of insulin dose, such that intensive management may be especially appropriate in their care. Patients with long life expectancy, without advanced diabetes complications or hypoglycemia unawareness may benefit from this management strategy.

Table 1.2 Adverse Effects of Intensive Diabetes Management

- If near-normal glycemia or euglycemia is achieved, the potential for hypoglycemia is increased.
- If hypoglycemia is more frequent, hypoglycemia unawareness can occur.
- Weight gain can occur.
- Diabetic ketoacidosis can occur if using continuous subcutaneous insulin infusion as pump malfunctions or cannula problems can interrupt insulin delivery.
- Patient may perceive not meeting goals as a personal failure.
- Patient may perceive that more personal time is spent on diabetes care.

INTENSIVE DIABETES MANAGEMENT

Intensive diabetes management is a mode of treatment the goal of which is eugly-cemia or near-normal glycemia. Achieving this goal involves the integration of several diabetes treatment components into the individual's lifestyle. These components include

- an individualized medication regimen
- frequent blood glucose monitoring
- CGM
- the use of pre- and postprandial SMBG data, blood glucose patterns and trends to meet individually defined treatment goals
- active adjustment of medication, food, and/or activity, based on blood glucose measurements
- active use of carbohydrate counting as a strategy to match food with insulin
- ongoing interaction between the individual with diabetes and the health care team
- assessment
  - education
  - medical care and treatment
  - emotional and psychological support
  - frequent objective assessment of glycemic control (A1c measurement)

In addition, a thorough understanding of diabetes and its management by all professional personnel involved in the daily care of this disease is crucial (Table 1.3).

Intensive diabetes management is the preferred therapeutic approach for many patients with diabetes (Table 1.4). This position is confirmed by the results of prospective studies, especially the DCCT, that show that lowering mean blood glucose levels and A1c near normal, reduces the development or worsening of the microvascular complications of diabetes. Glucose lowering in the intensive treatment arm of the DCCT was also associated with long-term benefit with regard to cardiovascular complications. The UKPDS and the Kumamoto study on intensive therapy in type 2 diabetes established essentially identical results in patients with type 2 diabetes.

It is clear that intensive diabetes management in women who are planning to become pregnant or who are pregnant lowers maternal morbidity and mortality to a level that matches the risk of women without diabetes. Maintenance of eug-lycemia ensures that the fetus is not exposed to an adverse maternal milieu. The

Table 1.3 Requirements for Intensive Diabetes Management

- Availability of experienced health care professionals
- Motivated patient
- Strong family support for children and adolescents
- Motivated parents and a health care team experienced in pediatric diabetes care

Table 1.4 Indications for Intensive Diabetes Management

- Otherwise healthy adults with either type 1 or type 2 diabetes
- Desire to avoid or lessen micro- and macrovascular complications
- Pregnancy in a woman with diabetes
- Any person who wishes to achieve near-normal glycemic control
- Hypoglycemia complicating conventional management
- Irregular lifestyle with insulin requirement
- Athletes having insulin requirement
- Cystic fibrosis
- Geriatric patient with type 2 diabetes experiencing insulin sensitivity, hypoglycemia unawareness, or defective counter regulations
- Patients who have had kidney transplantation for diabetic nephropathy

risk of peripartum complications and congenital malformations closely approaches that of the offspring of a mother without diabetes.

Most patients with type 1 diabetes will require multiple daily insulin injections or an insulin pump to achieve the goals of treatment. For patients with type 2 diabetes, successful intensified therapy (with goals similar to those in type 1 diabetes) may be possible with lifestyle interventions (regular physical exercise and careful medical nutrition therapy to lose weight). In patients with type 2 diabetes with greater degrees of insulin deficiency, oral glucose-lowering medications (biguanides, sulfonylureas, thiazolidinediones, glinides, alpha-glucosidase inhibitors, dipeptidyl peptidase IV inhibitors) singly or in combination, non-insulin injectable glucose-lowering medications (glucagon-like peptide-1 analogues, amylin analogues), and/or insulin are needed to achieve near-normal glycemia. The goals of therapy may necessarily be modified in some patients because of age, comorbid states, ability to adhere to a schedule of regular follow-up assessments, or other individual clinical situations that make the risks of intensified diabetes management greater than the benefits (Table 1.5). The balance between risk and benefit

Table 1.5 Contraindications to Intensive Diabetes Management

- Short life expectancy
- Lack of desire by the patient to implement intensive diabetes management
- Refusal to perform the technical tasks necessary for success and/or safety
- Refusal to agree to scheduled follow-up visits
- Social reasons
- Limited financial resources
- Inability to comprehend the techniques of implementation
- Presence of extensive end-stage microvascular complications that would make intensive diabetes management dangerous
- Blindness
- Chronic, irremediable autonomic neuropathic complications
- End-stage renal failure
- Any medical, social, or psychological problem that adversely affects the benefit-to-risk ratio

may be more delicate in the child without appropriate family support or in the elderly patient.

Intensive glycemic control as a goal is no longer limited to patients primarily in the outpatient setting. Numerous reports support the goal of near-normal blood glucose control in patients with diabetes admitted to a coronary care unit or undergoing open heart surgery. When intravenous insulin is used for glycemic control, morbidity and mortality are lowered. However, it is important to note that the NICE-SUGAR study, a large, international, randomized trial, found that intensive glucose control increased mortality among adults in the ICU: a blood glucose target of 180 mg or less per deciliter, resulted in lower mortality than did a target of 81 to 108 mg per deciliter. Other observations from intensive care units have been reported in patients without diabetes, showing that survival is enhanced by maintaining near-normal glycemia.

PHYSIOLOGICAL BASIS OF INTENSIVE MANAGEMENT METHODS

Intensive diabetes management attempts to normalize fuel metabolism by delivering insulin and/or oral diabetes medications to approximate normal physiology. Although the goal of completely normal physiology cannot be achieved with available methods, it is possible to improve glycemic control enough to have a dramatic impact on the risk of chronic complications.

NORMAL FUEL METABOLISM

Fuel metabolism is regulated by a complex system involving

- multiple tissues and organs
- intracellular enzyme systems to use nutrient fuels
- hormones and other regulatory factors to
  - distribute ingested nutrients to organs and tissues according to the needs for mechanical or chemical work and tissue growth or renewal
  - provide storage of excess nutrients as glycogen and fat
  - allow release of energy from storage depots as needed during periods of fasting or exercise

Carbohydrate Metabolism

Glucose is a major energy source for muscles and the brain. The brain is nearly totally dependent on glucose, whereas muscles also use fat and ketone bodies for fuel. The two main sources of circulating glucose are hepatic glucose production and ingested carbohydrate. After absorption of a meal is complete, glucose production by the liver supplies all the glucose needed for tissues such as the brain that do not store glucose. This is referred to as *basal glucose production* and is generally ~2 mg/kg body wt/min in adults. With increasing duration of a fast, as hepatic glycogen stores are exausted the relative contribution of gluconeogenesis to basal glucose production increases; however, normally about 50% of basal glucose production is from glycogenolysis; the rest is from gluconeogenesis.

Ingested carbohydrate is hydrolyzed into component sugars during intestinal digestion and monosaccharides are absorbed, producing a postprandial increase in blood glucose level that peaks 60–120 minutes after the meal. The magnitude and rate of increase in blood glucose are determined by many factors, including the size of the meal, its carbohydrate content, the physical state of the food (e.g., solid, liquid, cooked, raw), the presence of other nutrients (e.g., fat and fiber, which slow digestion), the amount of insulin, and the individual's sensitivity to insulin. The rate of gastric emptying also modulates postprandial blood glucose levels. These factors, in addition to the glycemic index and amount of ingested carbohydrate, have significant effects on glycemia.

Glucose is either oxidized for energy or stored as glycogen or fat. After ingestion of oral carbohydrate, 60–70% is stored, mostly as glycogen; the remainder is oxidized for immediate energy needs.

Protein Metabolism

Ingested protein is absorbed as amino acids, which may be used in three ways:

1. synthesis of new protein
2. oxidation to provide energy
3. conversion to glucose (gluconeogenesis)

During fasting, proteolysis and conversion of gluconeogenic amino acids to glucose prevent hypoglycemia. Alanine is the major amino acid substrate for hepatic gluconeogenesis; glutamine is the major amino aside substrate for renal gluconeogenesis. Branched-chain amino acids may be used for protein synthesis or oxidized for energy. They are the major donors of amino groups for synthesis of alanine, which can be readily converted to glucose.

Fat Metabolism

Fat is the major form of stored energy. Fat stored as triglyceride is converted to free fatty acids and glycerol by lipolysis. Free fatty acids from adipose tissue may be transported to muscle for oxidation. Oxidation of free fatty acids in the liver produces the ketone bodies acetoacetate and beta-hydroxybutyrate (referred to as *ketogenesis*). Synthesis of ketone bodies is, therefore, a stage in fat oxidation; they can be oxidized in extra-hepatic tissues to produce energy. Much of the ingested fat in a meal is efficiently stored in adipose tissue or muscle. Normally,

Table 1.6 Regulation of Fuel Metabolism by Hormones

	Insulin	Glucagon	Catecholamine	Cortisol	Growth Hormone
Glucose uptake	+	0	−	−	−
Gluconeogenesis	−	+	+	+	+
Glycogenolysis	−	+	+	+	+
Lipolysis	−	+	+	+	+
Ketogenesis	−	+	+	+	+

+, increases; −, decreases; 0, no effect.

only a small fraction of a glucose load is taken up by fat cells. In states of chronic excess nutrition, however, ingested fat is not oxidized and excess nutrients (glucose) are converted to fat and stored in adipose tissue. Elevated circulating free fatty acids from ingested fat or lipolysis blunt peripheral insulin action and slow the postabsorptive decrease in blood glucose.

REGULATION OF FUEL METABOLISM

Fuel metabolism is regulated by several hormones. The central nervous system (CNS) has an important role in this regulation, either through hormones or in other ways that are incompletely understood. The major hormones and their effects are summarized in Table 1.6 and discussed in more detail later in this chapter.

Insulin

Insulin is the major hypoglycemic hormone. It acts on liver, fat, and skeletal muscle to increase glucose uptake, oxidation and storage and to decrease glucose production. Insulin also inhibits lipolysis, and thereby limits the availability of fatty acids for oxidation and limits ketogenesis.

Insulin is secreted in two major patterns—basal and prandial. Basal secretion produces relatively constant, low plasma insulin levels that restrain lipolysis and glucose production. Abnormally low levels of basal insulin secretion result in markedly increased glucose production, lipolysis, and ketogenesis, causing hyperglycemia, hyperfattyacidemia, and ketosis. During exercise, skeletal muscle and other tissues require access to stored energy. Insulin secretion decreases to make stored energy available by allowing increased glucose production and lipolysis to occur. The blood glucose level is the dominant stimulus for insulin secretion. Beta cells of the pancreatic islet constantly monitor glucose levels so that insulin secretion is closely linked to changes in glycemia. Even small increases in blood glucose concentrations normally cause an increase in insulin secretion. Prandial insulin secretion rapidly increases to a level many times greater than basal levels. Higher postprandial insulin levels completely suppress hepatic glucose production and lipolysis, and stimulate uptake of ingested glucose by insulin-sensitive tissues.

Counterregulatory Hormones

Glucagon, catecholamines (epinephrine and norepinephrine), cortisol, and growth hormone are termed *counterregulatory hormones* because their actions are opposite to those of insulin. Together with insulin, they regulate metabolism under widely varying conditions. These hormones are often referred to as *stress hormones* because their levels in the circulation increase in response to stress. It has been suggested that this response is designed to provide the extra energy that may be needed to cope with stress. The concept of hypoglycemia-associated autonomic failure (HAAF) in diabetes posits that recent antecedent iatrogenic hypoglycemia causes both defective glucose counterregulation (by reducine the epinephrine response to falling glucose levels in the setting of an absent glucagon response) and hypoglycemia unawareness (by reducing the autonomic and the resulting neurogenic symptom responses) and thus a vicious cycle of recurrent hypoglycemia. Perhaps the most compelling support of HAAF is the finding that as little as

2–3 weeks of avoidance of hypoglycemia reverses hypoglycemia unawareness and improves the reduced epinephrine component of defective glucose counterregulation in most affected individuals.

Glucagon. Glucagon is the first line of defense against hypoglycemia in people who do not have diabetes. When blood glucose levels fall, the plasma glucagon concentration rapidly increases, and glucagon potently and rapidly stimulates hepatic glucose production by increasing glycogenolysis and gluconeogenesis. In type 1 diabetes, despite the loss of beta cell function, glucagon secretion by the pancreatic alpha cells persists. Glucagon secretion can promote hepatic glucogenesis inappropriate to ambient glucose elevations, in part responsible for fasting hyperglycemia and mediating the rise of glucose that occurs despite fasting or emesis when insulin levels are insufficient. On the other hand, appropriate glucagon responsiveness to hypoglycemia is lost among many persons with long-standing diabetes mellitus, espeically if their diabetes has been tightly controlled, resulting in the loss of this important defense mechanism against hypoglycemia.

Catecholamines. Catecholamines are produced at times of stress ("fight or flight") and also stimulate release of stored energy. Epinephrine stimulates glucose production and limits glucose utilization in insulin-sensitive tissues such as skeletal muscle. Catecholamines are the major defense against hypoglycemia in patients with type 1 diabetes who have lost their glucagon response to hypoglycemia. Hypoglycemia unawareness and sluggish recovery from hypoglycemia may occur when this defense is defective. Patients with hypoglycemia unawareness are at considerably increased risk for severe and prolonged hypoglycemia, and should embark on intensified glucose control only with great caution after a period of hypoglycemia avoidance and restoration of catecholamine responsiveness.

Cortisol. Secretion of this hormone also increases at times of stress. Its major effect is to stimulate gluconeogenesis; however, the onset of this effect is much slower than that of glucagon. The hyperglycemic response to cortisol is delayed for several hours. Consequently, cortisol is not effective in protecting against acute hypoglycemia. Cortisol also limits glucose utilization in several tissues including skeletal muscle.

Growth hormone. Growth hormone also has slow effects on glucose metabolism. A major surge of growth hormone secretion occurs during sleep and is responsible for an increase in insulin resistance in the early morning, termed the *dawn phenomenon.* Normally, a slight increase in insulin secretion compensates for the effects of nocturnal growth hormone secretion, but in diabetes the result may be morning hyperglycemia.

IMPLICATIONS FOR THERAPY

The most effective treatment regimens for diabetes attempt to replicate normal physiology. Important elements of treatment include

- a relatively constant low blood insulin level during fasting
- a rapid increase in blood insulin levels with meals, in an amount appropriate to the quantity and macronutrient content of food eaten

■ a decrease in insulin levels with vigorous and especially prolonged exercise or prolonged fasting

■ frequent blood glucose measurements and CGM to guide adjustments in insulin dose and other components of the regimen

Even the most complicated insulin regimen cannot account for all the conditions that influence blood glucose levels. Indeed, variable absorption of insulin from its subcutaneous injection site is one important factor contributing to blood glucose variation. Therefore, even the best methods currently available do not produce "perfect control." Patients with diabetes may adhere to every aspect of management and still have unexplained blood glucose variations. They should be counseled to expect some variability in blood glucose levels that may be difficult or impossible to account for. Nonetheless, meticulous attention to many small details greatly improves the control that can be achieved.

BIBLIOGRAPHY

Ahern J, Boland E, Doane R, Ahern J, Rose P, Vincent M, Tamborlane WV: Insulin pump therapy in pediatrics: a therapeutic alternative to safely lower HbA1c levels across all age groups. *Pediatric Diabetes* 3:10–15, 2002

American Diabetes Association: Standards of medical care in diabetes–2012. *Diabetes Care* 35 (Suppl. 1):S11–S63, 2012

Bode BW, Sabbah HT, Gross TM, Fredrickson LP, Davidson PC: Diabetes management in the new millennium using insulin pump therapy. *Diabetes Metab Res Rev* 18 (Suppl. 1):S14–S20, 2002

Cryer PE: Hypoglycemia-associated autonomic failure in diabetes. *Am J Physiol Endocrinol Metab* 281(6):E1115–E1121, 2001

Diabetes Control and Complications Trial (DCCT) Research Group: The effect of intensive treatment of diabetes on the development and progression of long-term complications in insulin-dependent diabetes mellitus. *N Engl J Med* 329:977–986, 1993

Diabetes Control and Complications Trial (DCCT) Research Group: Hypoglycemia in the Diabetes Control and Complications Trial. *Diabetes* 46:271–286, 1997

The Diabetes Control and Complications Trial/Epidemiology of Diabetes Interventions and Complications Research Group: Effect of intensive therapy on the microvascular complications of type 1 diabetes mellitus. *JAMA* 287:2563–2569, 2002

The Diabetes Control and Complications Trial/Epidemiology of Diabetes Interventions and Complications Research Group. Sustained effect of intensive treatment of type 1 diabetes mellitus on development and progression of diabetic nephropathy: the Epidemiology of Diabetes Interventions and Complications (EDIC) study. *JAMA* 22:290:2159–67, 2003

Gaede P, Vedel P, Larsen N, Jensen GV, Parving HH, Pedersen O: Multifactorial intervention and cardiovascular disease in patients with type 2 diabetes. *N Engl J Med* 348:383–393, 2003

Gray A, Raikou M, McGuire A, Fenn P, Stevens R, Cull C, Stratto I, Adler A, Holman R, Turner R: Cost effectiveness of an intensive blood glucose control policy in patients with type 2 diabetes: economic analysis alongside a randomised controlled trial (UKPDS 41): United Kingdom Prospective Diabetes Study Group. *BMJ* 320:1373–1378, 2000

Hirsch IB: Implementation of intensive diabetes therapy for IDDM. *Diabetes Reviews* 3:288–307, 1995

Hirsch IB: Insulin analogues. *N Engl J Med* 352:174–183, 2005

The Juvenile Diabetes Research Foundation Continuous Glucose Monitoring Study Group: Continuous glucose monitoring and intensive treatment of type 1 diabetes. *N Engl J Med* 359:1464–1476, 2008

Kitzmiller JL, Block JM, Brown FL, Catalano PM, Conway DL, Coustan DR, et al: Managing Preexisting Diabetes for Pregnancy: Summary of Evidence and Consensus Recommendations for Care. *Diabetes Care* 31:1060–1079, 2008

Lepore G, Dodesini AR, Nosari I, Trevisan R: Both continuous subcutaneous insulin infusion and a multiple daily insulin injection regimen with glargine as basal insulin are equally better than traditional multiple daily insulin injection treatment. *Diabetes Care* 26:1321–1322, 2003

Linkeschova R, Raoul M, Bott U, Berger M, Spraul M: Less severe hypoglycaemia, better metabolic control, and improved quality of life in type 1 diabetes mellitus with continuous subcutaneous insulin infusion (CSII) therapy: an observational study of 100 consecutive patients followed for a mean of 2 years. *Diabet Med* 19:746–751, 2002

Martin CL, Albers J, Herman WH, Cleary P, Waberski B, Greene DA, Stevens MJ, Feldman EL: Neuropathy among the Diabetes Control and Complications Trial cohort 8 years after trial completion. *Diabetes Care* 29:340–344, 2006

Mehta SN, Wolfsdorf JI. Contemporary management of patients with type 1 diabetes. *Endocrinol Metab Clin North Am.* 39:573-93, 2010

Nathan DM, Cleary PA, Backlund JY, Genuth SM, Lachin JM, Orchard TJ, Raskin P, Zinman B: Intensive diabetes treatment and cardiovascular disease in patients with type 1 diabetes. *N Engl J Med* 353:2643–2653, 2005

Nathan DM, Lachin J, Cleary P, Orchard T, Brillon DJ, Backlund JY, O'Leary DH, Genuth SM: Intensive diabetes therapy and carotid intima-media thickness in type 1 diabetes mellitus. *N Engl J Med* 348:2294–2303, 2003

Nathan DM, Zinman B, Cleary PA, Backlund JY, Genuth S, Miller R, et al. Modern-day clinical course of type 1 diabetes mellitus after 30 years' duration: the diabetes control and complications trial/epidemiology of diabetes interventions and complications and Pittsburgh epidemiology of diabetes complication experience (1983–2005). *Arch Intern Med* 27;169:1307–16, 2009

NICE-SUGAR Study Investigators: Intensive versus conventional glucose control in critically ill patients. *N Engl J Med.* 360:1283–1297, 2009

Ohkubo Y, Kishikawa H, Araki E, Miyata T, Isami S, Motoyoshi S, Kojima Y, Furuyoshi N, Shichiri M: The Kumamoto study: intensive insulin therapy prevents the progression of diabetic microvascular complications in Japanese patients with non-insulin-dependent diabetes mellitus: a randomized prospective 6-year study. *Diabetes Res Clin Pract* 28:103–117, 1995

Phillip M, Battelino T, Rodriguez H, Danne T, Kaufman F: Use of insulin pump therapy in the pediatric age group: consensus statement from the European Society for Paediatric Endocrinology, the Lawson Wilkins Pediatric Endocrine Society, and the International Society for Pediatric and Adolescent Diabetes, endorsed by the American Diabetes Association and the European Association for the Study of Diabetes. *Diabetes Care* 30:1653–1662, 2007

Reichard P, Nilsson BY, Rosenqvist U: The effect of long-term intensified insulin treatment on the development of microvascular complications of diabetes. *N Engl J Med* 329:304–309, 1993

Selvin E, Marinopolous S, Berkenblit G, Rami T, Brancati FL, Powe NR, Golden SH: Meta-analysis: glycosylated hemoglobin and cardiovascular disease in diabetes mellitus. *Ann Intern Med* 141:421–431, 2004

Skyler JS, Bergenstal R, Bonow RO, Buse J, Deedwania P, Gale EAM, Howard BV, Kirkman MS, Kosiborod M, Reaven P, Sherwin R: Intensive glycemic control and the prevention of cardiovascular events: implications of the ACCORD, ADVANCE, and VA diabetes trials: a position statement of the American Diabetes Association and a scientific statement of the American College of Cardiology Foundation and the American Heart Association. *Diabetes Care* 2009; 32: 187–192

Storlien LH, Baur LA, Kriketos AD, Pan DA, Cooney GJ, Jenkins AB, Calvert GD, Campbell LV: Dietary fats and insulin action. *Diabetologia* 39:621–631, 1996

Stratton IM, Adler AI, Neil HA, Matthews DR, Mansley SE, Cull CA, Hadden D, Turner RC, Holman RR: Association of glycemia with macrovascular and microvascular complications of type 2 diabetes (UKPDS 35): prospective observational study. *BMJ* 321:405–412, 2000

Turner RC, Cull CA, Frighi V, Holman RR: Glycemic control with diet, sulfonylurea, metformin, or insulin in patients with type 2 diabetes: progressive requirement for multiple therapies (UKPDS49). *JAMA* 281:2005–2012, 1999

UK Prospective Diabetes Study Group: Intensive blood glucose control with metformin on complications in overweight patients with type 2 diabetes (UKPDS 34). *Lancet* 352:854–865, 1998

UK Prospective Diabetes Study Group: Intensive blood glucose control with sulfonylurea or insulin compared with conventional treatment and risks of complications in patients with type 2 diabetes (UKPDS 33). *Lancet* 352:837–853, 1998

van den Berghe G, Wouters P, Weekers F, Verwaest C, Bruyninckx F, Schetz M, Vlasselaers D, Ferdinande P, Lauwers P, Bouillon, R: Intensive insulin therapy in the critically ill patients. *N Engl J Med* 345:1359–1367, 2001

Wake N, Hisashige A, Katayama T, Kishikawa H, Ohkubo Y, Sakai M, Araki E, Shichiri M: Cost-effectiveness of intensive insulin therapy for type 2 diabetes: a 10-year follow-up of the Kumamoto study. *Diabetes Res Clin Pract* 48:201–210, 2000

White NH, Clearly PA, Dahms W, Goldstein D, Malone J, Tamborlane WV: Beneficial effects of intensive therapy of diabetes during adolescence: outcomes after the conclusion of the Diabetes Control and Complications Trial (DCCT). *J Pediatr* 139:804–812, 2001

Zerr KJ, Furnary AP, Grunkemeier GL, Bookin S, Kanhere V, Starr A: Glucose control lowers the risk of wound infection in diabetics after open heart surgery. *Ann Thorac Surg* 63:356–361, 1997

The Team Approach

Highlights
The Team Approach

- Multidisciplinary team management is an effective and efficient alternative for the provision of the multidimensional care and support that is demanded by diabetes.
- Multidisciplinary team management provides the patient with
  - medical diagnosis and treatment
  - focused diabetes self-management education
  - medical nutrition therapy and nutrition management assistance
  - psychosocial evaluation and support
- Team management necessitates
  - identification of common treatment goals
  - shared decision making
  - open communication and ongoing collaboration
  - active involvement by all team members
- The treatment plan must be individualized and incorporate
  - medical priorities and concerns
  - the patient's abilities, willingness, readiness, and resources
- Intensive management of diabetes requires active participation by the patient and health care providers.
- Active patient participation in care requires the willingness to
  - become involved in daily self-care
  - acquire the skills necessary to make reasoned decisions
  - define the daily schedule and environment
  - implement the necessary treatment interventions
  - maintain frequent, open, and honest communication with health care providers
  - advocate for personal self care needs
- Health care provider responsibilities are to
  - establish treatment goals
  - inform and educate
  - negotiate needed lifestyle changes

- facilitate achievement of knowledgeable independence in self-care
- Effective team communication requires
  - common philosophy and message
  - common expectations
  - flexible professional boundaries
  - shared responsibility
  - an open approach to management interventions
- Patients must hear the same message from each member of the treatment team for any message to be heard.

The Team Approach

The American Diabetes Association (ADA) supports the position that intensive diabetes management should be considered for most patients with diabetes. Like that of many other chronic diseases, management of diabetes requires that lifestyle issues be addressed if the interventions are to be accepted and successfully integrated. However, few disorders demand such a high level of daily attention to behavioral issues and choices. Although most health care providers recognize the existence of these issues, objective analysis of current diabetes health care practices reveals a significant and continued discrepancy between this knowledge and actual practice patterns. The message *glycemic control matters* must be translated into individually defined health care choices and treatment decisions.

Multidisciplinary team management has become increasingly accepted as an effective and efficient alternative for providing the multidimensional care and support that diabetes demands. This approach emphasizes focused diabetes education, nutrition management, interventions that enhance physical fitness, and psychosocial support, all of which complement the traditional medical model approach that includes diagnosis and treatment. Comprehensive diabetes management by a multidisciplinary team does not obviate the need for or value of the solo medical practitioner. Instead, it illustrates the unique nature of diabetes management. Lack of time and multidimensional expertise are significant constraints in the health care system that currently cares for most individuals with diabetes. In the presence of irrefutable data that intensive diabetes management is beneficial, appropriate care can no longer be expected to occur in the context of two to four 10-minute medical management visits per year.

CONCEPT OF TEAM MANAGEMENT

Multidisciplinary team management encompasses a group of individuals from various disciplines who are focused on common health care goals. A team is a group of individuals with similar interests but different areas of professional expertise. As a group, they have a common purpose or focus. Each team member is responsible for contributing opinions and making decisions that support the common goals. The effectiveness of any team depends on the ability of team members to communicate and collaborate in the identification and achievement of their goals (Table 2.1).

Management of diabetes necessitates active involvement by both the patient and the health care providers. After the commitment to care has been made, a

Table 2.1 Factors That Influence Team Function

- Common goals and objectives
- Role expectations of each team member
- Decision-making process
- Communication patterns
- Leadership
- Accepted practice behaviors for team members (informally defined)

treatment plan can be created. Issues to consider when establishing a treatment plan include

- the patient's understanding of diabetes treatment and management
- ongoing assessment and treatment based on medical diagnosis and needs
- acquisition of technical skills, knowledge, and proficiency
- ongoing assessment of the management components and treatment approach
- recognition of the obstacles to appropriate self-care and development of intervention strategies to address them
- creation of a communication plan that facilitates ongoing interaction between the patient and the health care providers

The treatment plan must be individualized to the patient, taking into consideration medical priorities and giving ample attention to the patient's abilities as well as his or her willingness and readiness to carry out the defined interventions (Fig. 2.1). Knowledge of the need to make changes in health care behavior is, alone, often insufficient to motivate positive change. Thus, patient willingness and actual ability to carry out self-care behaviors must be evaluated on an ongoing basis.

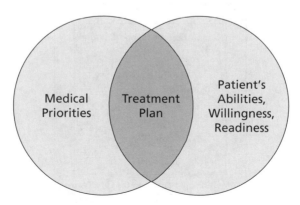

Figure 2.1 Treatment plan.

INTEGRATED DIABETES MANAGEMENT TEAM

The individual with diabetes is the central member of the diabetes health care team and requires training to assume primary responsibility for ongoing care. This individual is guided in self-care practices and management interventions by the multidisciplinary health care team. The patient's self-management efforts are further supported by nonprofessional individuals who play important roles in the patient's day-to-day life, such as spouses, significant others, parents, children, teachers, friends, and coworkers (Fig. 2.2). For this team to function effectively, each member must assume certain responsibilities. Team cohesion and consensus will determine the impact of treatment, both positive and negative, on glycemic outcome. As the central member of the diabetes management team, the patient must make the commitment to self-care (Table 2.2). Without this commitment, progress will be limited. After being made, this commitment is expanded and incorporates a willingness to become an active participant in health care. Active participation means

- defining the environment in which the diabetes care will occur
- establishing the daily schedule
- implementing the necessary treatment interventions
- acquiring the necessary skills to make reasoned decisions regarding treatment plan changes
- being willing to maintain frequent, open, and honest communication with the health care team

Ongoing care involves the integration of complex self-care techniques and subsequent alterations of lifestyle habits and patterns. Continued incorporation of self-care techniques enables patients to achieve increased flexibility in the management regimen and an increased sense of mastery over their disease.

Health care providers have the responsibility to inform and educate the patient about treatment options, work with the patient to establish treatment goals, and then to negotiate and promote needed lifestyle changes (Table 2.3). The

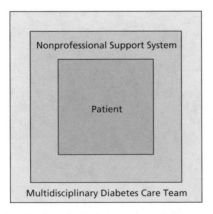

Figure 2.2 Integrated diabetes health care team.

Table 2.2 Patient Responsibilities

- Commit to intensive treatment
- Participate as an active member of the treatment team
- Make ongoing decisions regarding daily management
- Identify environmental factors affecting the treatment plan
- Advocate for personal self-care needs
- Communicate frequently and honestly with the diabetes care team about regimen preferences and treatment goals, fears about adverse consequences of intensive regimen, and/or concerns about implementation of regimen behaviors

goal of intervention is to facilitate the achievement of knowledgeable independence in self-care based on the individual's abilities. Ongoing communication (problem solving, feedback, and reality-based reinforcement) guides the patient's efforts. Patient education programs must incorporate

- technical skills training
- adjustment guidelines for variable diet, physical activity, and current glycemia
- problem-solving techniques
- guidance regarding both the prospective management of risks of intensified diabetes care and the need to monitor and manage diabetes comorbidities
- identification of interpersonal and practical supports that will enable patients to succeed in their efforts to intensify their care regimen

The health care team plays a vital role in the implementation of intensive diabetes management (Table 2.4). Before assisting patients with implementation of the treatment plan, however, health care providers must be realistic about their personal beliefs regarding the value of intensive diabetes treatment. Unless providers are knowledgeable and committed to the concept of intensive management and have access to the additional resources needed to ensure safe and effective treatment, their ability to assist patients in defining and/or achieving intensive treatment goals

Table 2.3 Health Care Provider Responsibilities

- Know the American Diabetes Association's (ADA's) Clinical Practice Recommendations
- Understand the scientific and clinical data on which ADA's Clinical Practice Recommendations are based
- Use ADA's Clinical Practice Recommendations to define and evaluate diabetes care delivery and practices
- Facilitate implementation of an effective treatment plan through ongoing education and communication
- Foster the development of "knowledgeable independence" in self-care practices
- Provide ongoing feedback and reinforcement
- Facilitate access to health care providers who are experienced in diabetes self-management and who are supportive of guided self-management

Table 2.4 Health Care Team Characteristics That Influence Success of Intensive Diabetes Management Efforts

- Belief in the benefits of intensive diabetes management
- Respect for other team members, including the patient
- Appreciation for the value of patient–health care provider collaboration in defining self-care behaviors and making management decisions
- Willingness to commit resources and effort to intensive management implementation
- Ability to provide or to access multidisciplinary education and health care expertise
- Understanding of the risks associated with intensive diabetes management
- Availability of 24-hour assistance for problem solving

will be compromised. Health care providers must also ensure that ADA's Clinical Practice Recommendations are met. Achieving this goal necessitates an awareness and use of the Clinical Practice Recommendations to define practice behaviors and health care delivery.

The availability of 24-hour access to health care providers who are knowledgeable about intensive diabetes self-management often can avert trips to emergency rooms and can prevent hospitalizations. If such health care provider availability does not exist, the risks associated with intensive management may outweigh the potential benefits and, thus, interfere with a patient's ability to achieve optimal glycemic control.

If the health care team is not readily available or adequately prepared with the additional knowledge, skills, and resources necessary to implement intensive diabetes management and/or is not committed to utilization of this form of therapy, it would be better to refer those patients who wish to intensify their management to centers that are prepared to undertake this endeavor. A collaborative relationship between the personnel at the referral center and the primary care provider is crucial to the success and effectiveness of the patient's treatment plan. This relationship is particularly important in view of the fact that the primary care provider is often the recipient of after-hours calls from patients.

ROLE DEFINITION

A clear understanding of the team goals, as well as the roles and responsibilities of individual team members, is a key requirement for a team to be successful. Each member's contribution to the team effort should be determined by his or her educational background, credentials, individual abilities, experience, interests, and overall goals of team operation. Typical roles and responsibilities for the physician, nurse, dietitian, and mental health professional members of the diabetes care team are listed in Table 2.5. Note that there is considerable overlap between roles, and few roles are exclusive.

The team's effectiveness will be influenced by the ability of its members to collaborate rather than to compete. Within the multidisciplinary framework, no team member operates in isolation. Instead, expertise and strengths are combined to enhance the delivery of comprehensive patient care. The addition of

---

Table 2.5 Typical Roles and Responsibilities of the Diabetes Care Team Members

- Role of the physician
  - Establish medical diagnosis and define treatment
  - Provide rationale for treatment
  - Collaborate with the patient and team to design and implement a treatment plan
  - Encourage the patient to work with the team to design and implement a treatment plan
  - Oversee total patient management
  - Provide patient/family support
- Role of the nurse manager/educator/clinician
  - Self-care assessment
  - Patient education: self-management skills, technical proficiency, compensatory adjustments, and problem solving
  - Family education/assessment
  - Interim contact: acute problem management, preventive care education, and blood glucose pattern review
  - Team effort coordination
  - Provide patient/family support
- Role of the dietitian
  - Nutrition assessment
  - Meal plan development
  - Specialized medical nutrition therapy
  - Interim contact: meal plan integration/modification, compensatory adjustments for variable food intake and/or exercise, and blood glucose pattern review
  - Provide patient/family support
- Role of mental health professional
  - Elicit and address patient/family concerns and fears about treatment regimen and possible adverse events
  - Identify treatment obstacles
  - Identify sources of support in the patient's environment that may compromise or enhance success of an intensive regimen
  - Provide patient/family support

---

these disciplines to the current medical model serves to extend the scope and availability of assessment, intervention, follow-up, and treatment for the individual with diabetes.

Comprehensive team management also can occur in settings where, through referral, a team is composed of members located at different sites or within separate facilities. For this approach to be effective, added emphasis must be placed on ongoing, accurate, and complete communication among the team members. Creativity and ingenuity can be used to facilitate the communication process by electronic transmissions, as well as verbal and written communication. Absence of specific health care team resources within a given facility should not be a deterrent to the use of a multidisciplinary approach to diabetes management. However, as with multidisciplinary teams that share the same venue, members of the treatment team must share common treatment goals and cooperate in treatment decisions to minimize confusion and conflict for the patient (see Team Communication).

In practice settings where a full complement of team members is not available and referral to a tertiary care center is not possible or is unacceptable, attempts still must be made to provide comprehensive education and care. Providers in this setting will need to become knowledgeable in all aspects of intensive management if they plan to provide comprehensive intensive diabetes care.

TEAM COMMUNICATION

Integrated team functioning requires the definition of a common philosophy regarding diabetes care practices and the development of a consistent treatment message and approach (Table 2.6). Patients must hear the same message from all members of the treatment team for any message to be heard. Conflicting or incongruent directives from providers confuse patients and interfere with the patient's willingness and/or ability to carry out the treatment recommendations.

Within treatment teams, role definitions and boundaries serve to define certain tasks. However, the complex nature of diabetes management necessitates flexibility in these boundaries, resulting in a blending of roles and sharing of responsibilities. Rigid boundaries surrounding professional disciplines often result in a territorial approach to patient care, which limits the team's ability to meet the patient's needs whenever any team member is absent. By maintaining openness regarding the interdependent working possibilities among team members, patients are more likely to receive comprehensive care.

Team meetings provide an opportunity for members to readily communicate with each other and to maintain a focused approach to their health care practices (Table 2.7). If held on a regular basis, team meetings facilitate review of individual patient problems and/or progress, facilitate identification of health care system obstacles and patient care trends, and provide the forum for active problem-solving. In this context, problem-solving and solution definition take on a multidisciplinary flavor, decreasing the chance for conflicts among the members of the treatment team. Team meetings also facilitate ongoing support among the health care providers, with the mental health professional often assisting other staff members to recognize behaviors or intervention styles that may be counterproductive to the achievement of treatment goals. In the absence of regularly scheduled team meetings, an alternative communication strategy among team members needs to be identified (i.e., e-mail or voicemail) to ensure that the messages received by patients are consistent and that patient care is comprehensive.

Table 2.6 Fostering Effective Team Communication

- Have a common philosophy and message
- Have common defined expectations
- Be flexible with regard to professional boundaries
- Share responsibility
- Have an open approach to management interventions

Table 2.7 Conducting Effective Team Meetings

- Maintain focus on common philosophy and goals
- Review patient progress and/or problems
- Identify individual patient behaviors that can be targeted by the team to enhance treatment efficacy
- Identify health care system or clinic trends
- Provide active, multidisciplinary problem solving and solution definition
- Establish intrateam support

FUNCTIONAL CONSIDERATIONS

Team management may necessitate a functional change in the hierarchy of patient care responsibility. Team members who are certified as diabetes educators (CDEs) by the National Certification Board for Diabetes Educators, as well as those who are Board-Certified Advanced Diabetes Managers (BC-ADMs) under the joint sponsorship of the American Nurses Credentialing Center (ANCC) and the American Association of Diabetes Educators (AADE), are expected to function at a specialist level. Certification provides an objective means of defining and evaluating knowledge and practice behaviors. As certified practitioners, these health care professionals assume a portion of the legal responsibility for education practices and diabetes care delivery. In addition, the establishment of the National Standards for Diabetes Self-Management Education, which are used by the American Diabetes Association's (ADA) Education Recognition Program and the American Association of Diabetes Educators' (AADE) Diabetes Education Accreditation Program to identify quality diabetes education programs, has further defined the level of intervention and care expected of these practitioners and the programs they administer.

Access to health care systems and health care provider practices that offer team management continues to be limited, often because of fiscal constraints. However, in situations in which practices and/or procedures formerly performed by the physician become a routine and accepted part of the nonphysician provider's role, the patient is afforded more comprehensive support. Acceptance of this expanded role brings the expectation that nonphysician practitioners will be responsible, at least in part, for treatment assessment, direction, decisions, interventions, and evaluation. The conduct of these activities is guided by a common understanding of the expected outcomes along with written standardized procedures and educational interventions with stated goals, objectives, content, and evaluation.

BIBLIOGRAPHY

American Association of Diabetes Educators: The scope of practice, standards of practice and standards of professional performance for diabetes educators. http://www.diabeteseducator.org/export/sites/aade/_resources/pdf/research/ScopeStandards_Final2_1_11.pdf

American Association of Diabetes Educators: *The Art and Science of Diabetes Self-Management Education: A Desk Reference for Healthcare Professionals*. Chicago, American Association of Diabetes Educators, 2006

American Diabetes Association: *Medical Management of Type 1 Diabetes*. 5th ed. Kaufman F, Ed. Alexandria, VA, American Diabetes Association, 2008

American Diabetes Association: *Medical Management of Type 2 Diabetes*. 6th ed. Burant C, Ed. Alexandria, VA, American Diabetes Association, 2008

American Diabetes Association: Standards of Medical Care in Diabetes—2012. *Diabetes Care* 35:S11–S63, 2012

Anderson D, Christison-Lagay J: Diabetes self-management in a community health center: improving health behaviors and clinical outcomes for underserved patients. *Clinical Diabetes* 26:22–27, 2008

Brink SJ, Miller M, Moltz K: Education and multidisciplinary team care concepts for pediatric and adolescent diabetes mellitus. *Journal of Pediatric Endocrinology & Metabolism* 15:1113–1130, 2002

California Diabetes Program: Diabetes Team Care Toolkit, 2007: http://www.cal-diabetes.org/content_display.cfm?contentID=422

California Medi-Cal Type 2 Diabetes Study Group: Closing the gap: effect of diabetes case management on glycemic control among low-income ethnic minority populations. *Diabetes Care* 27:95–103, 2004

Caravalho JY, Saylor CR: An evaluation of a nurse case-managed program for children with diabetes. *Pediatr Nurs* 26:296–300, 328, 2000

Davidson MB: Effect of nurse-directed diabetes care in a minority population. *Diabetes Care* 26:2281–2287, 2003

Diabetes Control and Complications Trial (DCCT) Study Group: The effect of intensive treatment of diabetes on the development and progression of long-term complications in insulin-dependent diabetes mellitus. *N Engl J Med* 329:977–986, 1993

Franz MJ, Callahan T, Castle G: Changing roles: educators and clinicians. *Clinical Diabetes* 12:53–54, 1994

Funnell MM, Brown TL, Childs BP, Haas LB, Hosey GM, Jensen B, Maryniuk M, Peyrot M, Piette JD, Reader D, Siminerio LM, Weinger K, Weiss MA: National standards for diabetes self-management education. *Diabetes Care* 31:S97–S104, 2008

Glasgow RE, Hiss RG, Anderson RM, Friedman NM, Hayward RA, Marrero DG, Taylor CB, Vinicor F: Report of the Health Care Delivery Work Group: behavioral research related to the establishment of a chronic disease model for diabetes care. *Diabetes Care* 24:124–130, 2001

Goldhaber-Fiebert JD, Goldhaber-Fiebert SN, Tristán ML, Nathan DM: Randomized controlled community-based nutrition and exercise intervention improves glycemia and cardiovascular risk factors in type 2 diabetic patients in rural Costa Rica. *Diabetes Care* 26:24–29, 2003

Hirsch IB: The status of the diabetes team. *Clinical Diabetes* 16:145–146, 1998

Lawson ML, Frank MR, Fry MK, Perlman K, Sochett EB, Daneman D: Intensive diabetes management in adolescents with type 1 diabetes: the importance of intensive follow-up. *J Pediatr Endocrinol Metab* 13:79–84, 2000

Leicher SB, Dreelin E, Moore S: Integration of clinical psychology in the comprehensive diabetes care team. *Clinical Diabetes* 22:129–131, 2004

Lorenz RA, Bubb J, Davis D, Jacobson A, Jannasch K, Kramer J, Lipps J, Schlundt D: Changing behavior: practical lessons from the Diabetes Control and Complications Trial. *Diabetes Care* 19:648–652, 1996

National Diabetes Education Program, National Institutes of Health. Redesigning the Heath Care Team: Diabetes Prevention and Lifelong Management. Bethesda, Maryland: U.S. Department of Health and Human Services, 2011

Philis-Tsimikas A, Walker C, Rivard L, Talavera G, Reimann J, Salmon M, Araujo, R: Improvement in diabetes care of underinsured patients enrolled in Project Dulce: a community-based, culturally appropriate, nurse case management and peer education diabetes care model. *Diabetes Care* 27:110–115, 2004

Renders CM, Valk GD, Griffin SJ, Wagner EH, van Eijk JT, Assendelft WJJ: Interventions to improve the management of diabetes in primary care, outpatient, and community settings: a systematic review. *Diabetes Care* 24:1821–1833, 2001

Rubin, R: Facilitating self-care in people with diabetes. *Diabetes Spectrum* 14:55–57, 2001

UK Prospective Diabetes Study Group: Intensive blood glucose control with sulfonylureas or insulin compared with conventional treatment and risk of complications in patients with type 2 diabetes. *Lancet* 352:837–853, 1998

University of California San Diego Diabetes Control and Complications Trial (DCCT) Team: Blended roles, shared responsibilities: DCCT nurses and dietitians. *Diabetes Spectrum* 7:272–275, 1994

Wagner EH: The role of patient care teams in chronic disease management. *BMJ* 320:569–572, 2000

Yale University Diabetes Control and Complications Trial (DCCT) Group: Weekly meetings focus team efforts. *Diabetes Spectrum* 7:77–78, 1994

Diabetes Self-Management Education

Highlights
Diabetes Self-Management
Education

- The patient using intensive diabetes management must translate new information and skills into behavior change. Each interaction with the patient is an opportunity for the health care provider to teach, reinforce, and encourage. The team approach is best exemplified when information is consistent among team members.

- The patient's readiness to learn new information is a necessary component of any negotiated education plan. The individual will be most receptive when the education is relevant to his or her current needs. In addition, eliciting the patient's commitment to behavior change is another integral component of any education program.

- Educational assessment includes information about the patient's knowledge, skills, attitudes, and current diabetes care behaviors. The patient must possess a basic level of understanding before learning the more sophisticated aspects of intensive diabetes self-management.

- Education is communication and requires careful planning and delivery of pertinent information. Classes should be sequenced to build on existing knowledge. Teaching methods include the use of print and audiovisual media. These items must be content-appropriate, readable, and culturally sensitive.

- Intensive diabetes management requires active patient involvement and problem solving. As part of their education, some individuals may need assistance in actively participating in their care.

- Evaluating the success of patient education can be practical and quick. By using a series of "what if" questions, the educator is able to assess the patient's problem-solving abilities.

- Recording key aspects of the education experience allows diabetes educators to share information with primary care and referring physicians and other health care providers.

Diabetes Self-Management Education

As the Diabetes Control and Complications Trial (DCCT) demonstrated, diabetes self-management education is integral to the success of an intensive management program. Patients embarking on the road to glycemic control must not only understand the complexities of diabetes and perform the necessary technical skills, but also must believe in the management strategies and have confidence in their abilities. Intensive management requires patients to assume an active role in clinical decisions on a daily basis. To do this safely and effectively, patients need a supportive, knowledgeable, and accessible professional health care team.

Diabetes self-management education is successful when patients are able to translate the information and skills into behavior change. Consequently, diabetes education is more than a lecture or two on how to control the disease. Instead, it is an ongoing program of assessment, instruction, support, negotiation, and evaluation delivered by a team of diabetes professionals.

INTEGRATION OF THE TEAM APPROACH

A coordinated team of professionals provides depth to the patient's diabetes self-management education. The physician, nurse manager/educator/clinician, dietitian, and mental health professional, as well as the pharmacist and exercise physiologist, all contribute particular skills and focus. The physician may create a team by referring to a community-based patient education program or to local diabetes educators. The American Diabetes Association (ADA) and the American Association of Diabetes Educators (AADE) maintain lists of nationally recognized or accredited education programs. Additionally, the American Association of Diabetes Educators (AADE) assists in locating local diabetes educators. The National Certification Board for Diabetes Educators keeps a roster of certified diabetes educators.

Diabetes education should never stand alone. Instead, it is a component of the care and management of the patient with diabetes. All members of the treatment team are teachers. Each contact with the patient is an opportunity to teach, reinforce, or evaluate the effect of teaching.

Information must be consistent across professionals. This consistency allows the patient to develop the necessary trust in the management plan and in the health care providers. Educational materials must also be consistent in content. Consequently, each team member should know what the others are teaching.

31

Table 3.1 Basic Facts for the Candidate for Intensive Diabetes Management

- Medication: insulin action/insulin regimens; amylin analog
- Rationale for self-monitoring of blood glucose: frequency of checking, goals, patterns
- A1C: testing frequency, goals
- Nutrition management
  - Healthy food choices
  - Role of major nutrients: effect on blood glucose levels
  - Carbohydrate counting
  - Sick-day management
  - Label reading
  - Dining out/convenience foods
- Effect of exercise
- Interaction of exercise, nutrition, and medication
- Hypoglycemia: causes, treatment, prevention
- Glucagon
- Identifying the dawn phenomenon
- Hyperglycemia: causes, treatment, prevention
- Ketoacidosis: causes, treatment, prevention
- Complications: causes, symptoms, prevention, monitoring
- Effect of daily living on diabetes control
  - Alcohol and other drugs/drug interactions
  - Tobacco
  - Work schedules
  - Traveling
  - Illness/medications and control
- Individual's evaluation of his or her efforts

DIABETES CONTINUING EDUCATION

Diabetes information should be taught with the understanding that learning about and adjusting to the disease is an ongoing process. One class, or a series of classes, at diagnosis does not confer lifelong "immunity." Instead, education should be viewed as a treatment that requires periodic boosters and lifelong learning.

Patients vary in their willingness or readiness to learn. There are times when learner readiness is high: when new research findings are released, when new medications are available, when complications occur, and when developmental changes arise. These are times for the educator to capitalize on these "teachable moments" when the patient's motivation and interest are at a peak.

Ongoing diabetes self-management support (DSMS) also helps people with diabetes maintain effective self-management throughout a lifetime of diabetes as they face new challenges and as treatment advances become available. Diabetes Self Management Education (DSME) helps patients optimize metabolic control, prevent and manage complications, and maximize quality of life in a cost-effective manner.

DSME and DSMS are the on-going processes of facilitating the knowledge, skill, and ability necessary for self-care. This process incorporates the needs, goals,

Table 3.2 Eliciting the Patient's Beliefs

- What has been your experience with chronic health problems?
- How do you usually deal with success and failure?
- How has your diabetes affected your family?
- What worries or concerns you most about having diabetes?
- How do you typically learn new things?
- What one thing would you tell someone newly diagnosed with diabetes?
- What is the hardest part of diabetes management?
- What do you hope intensive diabetes management will do for you?
- How will you know if intensive diabetes management has been effective?

and life experiences of the person with diabetes. The overall objectives of DSME and DSMS are to support informed decision-making, self-care behaviors, problem-solving, and active collaboration with the health care team to improve clinical outcomes, health status, and quality of life in a cost-effective manner.

ASSESSMENT

The first step in developing an individualized education plan is to gather information about the patient's current knowledge, skills, attitudes, behaviors, and environment. Because intensive management is so dependent on the patient's involvement and decision making, certain basic facts and skills are necessary. Table 3.1 lists the prerequisite information for patients entering an intensive management program. In addition to having this prerequisite information, the patient must accurately and safely perform certain self-management skills. These skills include

- using a blood glucose meter or continuous glucose sensing device,
- troubleshooting problems with glucose measurements,
- testing urine or blood ketones,
- record keeping or data management,
- preparing and delivering insulin, and
- caring for the feet.

A careful educational assessment includes

- **Personal and socioeconomic information:** age; developmental stage; level of formal education; family composition; significant others; cultural, religious, and ethnic factors; resources; health insurance; and transportation
- **Diabetes information:** type and duration of diabetes, current and previous management approaches, acute and chronic complications, previous diabetes education, and successes and problems with adherence
- **Other medical information:** height, weight, blood pressure, pertinent laboratory values (e.g., blood glucose, A1c, estimated average glucose (eAG) lipids, microalbumin), other illnesses, other medications, general health status, visual and hearing acuity, and motor skills

Table 3.3 Qualities and Competencies of the Teacher

- Has a knowledge base that is current and extensive
- Holds a personal belief that patients can learn
- Is empathetic
- Is genuine
- Is adaptable: flexible in using a variety of teaching approaches
- Has a sense of humor
- Is able to
  - individualize information
  - encourage questions
  - allow adequate time for patients to answer
  - use clear, simple, concrete explanations
  - sequence educational topics
  - involve others as needed
  - repeat and reinforce facts
  - provide for reflection and review of content
  - evaluate understanding
  - provide focused and timely feedback

- **Lifestyle factors:** use of alcohol, tobacco, or other social drugs; physical activity; stressors; occupation; recreation; and social support systems
- **Nutrition information:** meal and snack times, locations, and typical foods; food preferences and intolerances; previous experience with "diets"; and previous nutrition education
- **Education factors:** learning style, literacy, native language, readiness to learn, decision-making skills, health information seeking behaviors, technology preferences, health beliefs (e.g., locus of control, confidence, experience with other chronic illnesses, coping patterns, fears, concerns [Table 3.2]), ability/willingness to seek help, expectations of and capacity to deal with failure, assertiveness skills, organizational skills, response to an education plan, and motivators or barriers

INSTRUCTION

ENVIRONMENT

The learning environment includes not only the physical facility, but also characteristics of the instructor who facilitates the learning. To help the patient focus on the content, the location should be quiet, with adequate lighting, and free from distractions. Such attention to the environment decreases the cognitive load to efficient learning. Qualities of the teacher that promote learning are included in Table 3.3.

The educator must draw from an extensive knowledge base while translating this knowledge into language understandable to the learner/patient. Furthermore, the educator must be able to adjust an educational agenda to meet the learner's needs. For example, the educator may have determined that the patient should hear about different insulin programs, whereas the patient may want to learn about counting carbohydrates. Adult learners will always be focused on what the education encounter will mean to them. The educator is most successful when able to adapt to changes in the teaching agenda.

Education is a process of communication and reception of information. Throughout the education session, the educator assesses the learner's understanding. By asking the patient to restate the information or to use the information to solve a problem, the educator is able to evaluate learning.

PLANNING

As the assessment proceeds, the educator will identify topics and teaching approaches that are most appropriate for the patient. Shared goal setting is important. The plan for the education program becomes a negotiation between the teacher and learner. Although it is the educator's responsibility to identify knowledge deficits, it is the learner's job to provide an accurate medical and educational history and to acknowledge what must be learned to safely undertake intensive management.

Often, the patient doesn't know what he or she needs to know and may be resistant to new information. The educator's job is to gently challenge the patient's knowledge while presenting new information. The educator may need to remind the patient that medical knowledge about diabetes changes rapidly and old information is being replaced with new ways of handling the disease.

The educator's job is to engage the patient/learner in the education by building trust and listening to the learner's needs. The patient is more likely to remain interested when the content is meaningful and is consistent with what the patient already knows. Strategies to maintain interest include using interactive teaching approaches and incorporating time for review and reflection of new content.

CONTENT

Topics especially pertinent for the patient implementing intensive diabetes management include

- nutritional guidelines and the effect of food on glycemic control,
- insulin action and dosage adjustment,
- impact of exercise on blood glucose control,
- monitoring,
- management of acute complications,
- prevention and detection of chronic complications,
- behavior change strategies, and
- problem solving.

A comprehensive curriculum list is included in Table 3.4.

SEQUENCING OF CLASSES

There is far too much information on intensive management to deliver in one session. Effective diabetes education occurs over several contacts with the patient. The most meaningful education sessions build on the patient's existing knowledge and on content from previous sessions. For instance, one session may be devoted to

Table 3.4 Curriculum for Intensive Management

- Diabetes overview and review
  - DCCT results: long-term control and benefits
  - Benefits, risks, and management options for improving glucose control
- Stress and psychosocial adjustment
  - Effect of stress on control
  - Identifying stressors
  - Anticipating stress
  - Problem solving: stress management techniques
- Family involvement and social support
  - Sharing diabetes care: when and how
  - Seeking help
  - Joining support groups
  - Doing volunteer work
- Nutrition
  - Role of nutrients
  - Glycemic impact
  - Label reading
  - Advanced carbohydrate counting or other system
  - Alcohol: effect and use
  - Dining out/Cooking in (adapting recipes)
  - Problem solving: evaluating effect of food adjustments/changes
- Exercise and activity
  - Effect of exercise
  - Exercise physiology
  - Prolonged effect, late post-exercise hypoglycemia
  - Planning pre-exercise food or insulin
  - Problem solving: evaluating effect of exercise
- Diabetes medication
  - Insulin: preparation, injection, storage, site selection
  - Insulin delivery systems: technical training for use of pens and pumps
  - Problem solving: insulin dose changes
    - Using results of monitoring to evaluate blood glucose patterns and variability
    - Basal changes
    - Bolus changes (i.e., algorithms)
    - Supplemental doses or sensitivity factors
    - Evaluating and verifying the effect of dose adjustment
    - When to call the diabetes team
  - Pramlintide: preparation, dosing, injection, storage, site selection, side-effects
- Monitoring
  - Blood glucose meter use: technique, meter care, troubleshooting
  - Fingerstick or alternative site technique, care of skin
  - Continuous glucose monitoring (when to use, how to use; interpreting results)
  - Record keeping and data management
  - Understanding and using blood glucose results
  - Testing at unusual times to gather information
  - When to test urine or blood ketones, and interpretation of results
  - Relationships among nutrition, exercise, medication, and blood glucose levels
  - Effect of daily variability
  - Effect of unusual days
    - Travel
    - Varying work schedules
  - Anticipating changes and making adjustments

Table 3.4 (*Continued*)

- Prevention, detection, and treatment of acute complications
  - Identifying symptoms of hypoglycemia
  - How symptoms may change as glycemic control improves
  - Glucagon: who to train, precautions
  - Dawn phenomenon: recognizing and managing
  - Symptoms of hyperglycemia and its management
  - Diabetic ketoacidosis
- Prevention, detection, and treatment of chronic complications
  - Detection of problems: routine health follow-up and diabetes-specific follow-up
  - Effect of intensification on existing complications
  - Foot, skin, and dental care
    - Injection sites: more frequent injections
    - Prevention of infections
    - Dental prophylaxis
- Behavior change strategies, goal setting, negotiation skills, and problem solving
  - Decision-making skills
  - Problem-solving approaches
  - Interacting with diabetes team
- Preconception, pregnancy, and postpartum management
- Use of health care systems and community resources
  - Creating a diabetes management team
  - Financial impact and cost-saving strategies for intensive diabetes management

a discussion about insulin regimens, the interpretation of blood glucose results, and record keeping. The next session may focus on problem solving by reviewing blood glucose records and discussing and demonstrating insulin adjustment techniques.

APPROACHES/STRATEGIES

Adults learn best when the information is immediately useful and relevant. Thus, teaching a patient to implement an intensive management plan must include enough time to practice the decision making required and focus on information needed to implement the treatment plan. For example, if the patient will be using an algorithm to adjust insulin doses, then the educator must plan for opportunities to practice using that algorithm.

The educator should have a repertoire of real-life examples to use when teaching. Most individuals need help to develop the judgment and problem solving needed to make diabetes decisions. Consider, for instance, what a patient must evaluate in choosing an insulin dose before a meal. How much carbohydrate will be consumed? What is the current blood glucose level? How far from target is the blood glucose level? What range of insulin doses tends to work for this mealtime? What will the exercise level be in the next couple of hours? How long should the time between injection and meal be? Working through several examples with the patient allows the educator to model decision making. Decision making and problem solving are skills acquired and improved through practice. Mistakes are part of the learning process. The educator must create opportunities

Table 3.5 Sample Worksheet for Intensive Diabetes Management

Goals for Intensive Blood Glucose Control

	ADA guidelines	*Personal goals*
Preprandial plasma glucose	70–130 mg/dl (3.9–7.2 mmol/l)	
Peak postprandial glucose	<180 mg/dl (<10.0 mmol/l)	
A1C	<7%	

Basal Insulin

Time	*Type*	*Dose*

Bolus Insulin

Time	*Type*	*Dose*	*Carbohydrate Amount*

Correction Insulin Dose: _____ units for every _____ mg/dl blood glucose

for practice and an environment where errors and misjudgments are used to learn, not criticize.

Other approaches include using print, audiovisual, and web-based materials. Many excellent materials are available from manufacturers of diabetes supplies. However, they must be individually evaluated for appropriate content, readability, and cultural sensitivity. Interactive educational materials—for example, computer programs, food models, self-instructional materials, and games—add variety to the education program and enhance learner engagement in the process. A sample patient education handout is provided in Table 3.5.

Regardless of the methodology for instruction, one of the most effective approaches to encouraging adherence is simple: Provide the literate patient with clear, written instructions. Patients generally remember very little from their time with the physician or educator. Written instructions can be the educator's most practical tool.

Table 3.6 Verifying the Patient's Commitment

- How effective do you think this treatment will be for you?
- What part of the plan may be hard for you?
- Are you concerned about the time or expense?
- How will you know if the plan is working?
- How certain are you that you can do this?
- What makes you certain or uncertain?
- If now is not the right time for you to begin, when will the time be right?

MOTIVATION AND SUPPORT

The process of patient education is intimately connected to behavior change. The educator should assess how the patient will use or transfer the information to action. Simply asking the patient, "How will you try this at home?" or "What things will be easy/hard to do?" will often alert the educator to potential difficulties in adherence. Some questions to elicit the patient's commitment to behavior change are listed in Table 3.6.

ACTION PLANNING

Some patients have adequate diabetes knowledge and wish to participate in their care, but lack the assertive communication or negotiation skills needed. They may feel intimidated by the health care professional or by the system. Yet, patient involvement in treatment decisions is important for the individual on an intensive management program. Because the patient will direct so much of the daily management, his or her commitment to the plan is essential.

Table 3.7 Providing Reflection and Review of Educational Content

- What are the three most important points?
- What questions do you still have?
- What did you find most interesting?
- What did you find most difficult?
- How would you summarize this content?
- How could you learn more about this topic?
- What did you learn that was new to you?
- What do you want always to remember?
- How does this content relate to something you already know?
- What will help you remember this material?
- What did you find most surprising?
- What will be the hardest thing to remember?
- How will you use what you learned today?
- What content will make the most difference for you?

Table 3.8 Evaluating Learning and Problem Solving

- What would you do if
  - you gave yourself insulin and your restaurant meal was late?
  - you were supposed to take lispro insulin before a meal, but your blood glucose level was 40 mg/dl?
  - you were planning to play tennis 1 hour after lunch?
  - you awakened with nausea and did not feel like eating?
  - your blood glucose results did not coincide with how you felt?
- How would you adjust your insulin for extra food or exercise?
- What would you tell your doctor if you thought that the plan was not working?
- How will you adjust your management plan for special occasions and parties?

The educator may assess commitment and confidence with a simple rating tool. After developing an action plan with the patient, the educator asks the patient to rate how confident he or she feels in following the plan. The patient rates confidence on a scale of 1 to 10 (1 being not at all confident; 10 being highly confident). The educator then explores what supports the chosen rating and what is preventing a higher rating. Such exploration reveals motivators or supports as well as barriers to behavior change.

The educator may find that the patient actually needs assistance in communicating his or her needs to the physician. The patient's education plan may include tips on how to participate actively in the treatment plan.

EVALUATION

Often in a busy practice, patient education amounts to nothing more than the professional relaying information, with very little time directed at assessing how the information is received and implemented. Whether provided in the physician's office or in a formal classroom education setting, evaluating the success of patient education can be quick and easy.

Tests and quizzes have a place in some education programs. However, the adult learner will remember information that is immediately useful. Education sessions should include sufficient time for reflection on the material discussed. Questions to promote reflection and review are listed in Table 3.7. Using a series of "what if" questions allows the educator not only to assess level of knowledge but also to determine problem-solving abilities. A sample of such questions is provided in Table 3.8.

DOCUMENTATION

The diabetes educator is obligated to completely document the education process from assessment through evaluation. Checklists and documentation forms may be created to assist the educator in this task. Sample forms are provided in the section on Education Recognition Program at http://professional.diabetes.org. To provide continuity and consistency and to facilitate the team approach, the educator, in addition to documenting the medical record, should also provide follow-up information to the referring physician or prescriber.

CONCLUSION

Patient education is integral to the success of intensifying the individual's diabetes management. The patient must be skilled and knowledgeable to participate fully and successfully in the decisions about daily self-care. The physician, diabetes educators, and other professionals must form a unified teaching team to ensure that the patient receives consistent and accurate information. Providing diabetes self-management education requires attention to patient assessment, individualized instruction, and evaluation of patient response.

BIBLIOGRAPHY

American Association of Diabetes Educators (AADE): *The Art and Science of Diabetes Self-Management Education: A Desk Reference for Healthcare Professionals*, 2nd Edition. Chicago, IL, AADE, 2011

American Diabetes Association: *Medical Management of Type 1 Diabetes*. 5th ed. Kaufman F, Ed. Alexandria, VA, American Diabetes Association, 2008

Anderson B, Funnel M: *The Art of Empowerment*. Alexandria, VA, American Diabetes Association, 2000

Bodenheimer T, Davis C, Holman H: Helping patients adopt healthier behaviors. *Clinical Diabetes* 25(2):66–70, 2007

Boren SA, Fitzner AK, Panhalkar PS, Specker J: Costs and benefits associated with diabetes education: A review of the literature. *The Diabetes Educator* 31(1):72–96, 2009

Childs B, Cypress M, Spollett G (Eds.): *Complete Nurse's Guide to Diabetes Care*. Alexandria, VA, American Diabetes Association, 2005

Dick W, Carey L, Carey JO: *The Systematic Design of Instruction*. 6th ed. Boston, MA, Pearson, 2005

Duncan I, Ahmed T, Li Q, Stetson B, Ruggiero L, Burton K, Rosenthal D, Fitzner K: Assessing the value of the diabetes educator. *The Diabetes Educator:* 37(5): 638-657, 2011

Funnell MM, Brown TL, Childs BP, Haas LB, Hosey GM, Jensen B, Maryniuk M, Peyrot M, Piette JD, Reader D, Siminerio LM, Weinger K, Weiss MA.: National standards for diabetes self-management education. *Diabetes Care* 34 (Suppl 1):S89–96, 2011

Gardner, H: *Multiple Intelligences: New Horizons*. New York, NY, Perseus Books Group, 2006

Gary TL, Genkinger JM, Guallar E, Peyrot M, Brancati FL: Meta-analysis of randomized educational and behavioral interventions in type 2 diabetes. *The Diabetes Educator* 29(3):488–501, 2003

King EB, Schlundt DG, Pichert JW, Kinzer CK, Backer BA: Improving the skills of health professionals in engaging patients in diabetes-related problem solving. *The Journal of Continuing Education in the Health Professions* 22(2):94–102, 2002

Mensing C: Comparing the processes: Accreditation and recognition. *Diabetes Spectrum* 23(1):65–78, 2010

Norris SL, Lau J, Smith SJ, Schmid CH, Engelgau MM: Self-management education for adults with type 2 diabetes: a meta-analysis of the effect on glycemic control. *Diabetes Care* 25(7):1159–1171, 2002

Rollnick S, Miller WR, Butler CC: *Motivational Interviewing in Health Care*. New York, NY, Guilford Press, 2008

Skyler JS, Ponder S, Kruger DF, Matheson D, Parkin C: Is there a place for insulin pump therapy in your practice? *Clinical Diabetes* 25:50–56, 2007

Sousa DA: *How the Brain Learns*. 3rd ed. Thousand Oaks, CA, Corwin Press, 2006

Psychosocial Issues

Highlights
Psychosocial Issues

■ Patients and their support team should be empowered, educated, and willing to accept responsibility for the increased self-care behaviors and lifestyle changes required by intensive diabetes management. Patient success with self-care behaviors and willingness to collaborate in treatment decisions are good indicators of future success with an intensive management plan.

■ Before intensification of diabetes management begins
  • patient self-management skills should be evaluated and training provided regarding skill deficits to establish competence with self-care
  • medical or psychological conditions that impair a patient's ability to make, evaluate, or communicate treatment decisions should be identified so that the necessary psychosocial supports and safeguards can be put in place

■ Psychosocial support is crucial to success with intensive diabetes management and must be ongoing. Support can come from health care providers, family members, and diabetes-specific or community support groups.

■ Patients are more likely to succeed with self-care regimens that are responsive to lifestyle needs and do not present an overwhelming burden. To support behavior change, self-care behaviors should be taught, monitored for mastery and effectiveness, and modified in an ongoing fashion. However, lapses in self-care behaviors should be expected as a routine part of care. Lifestyle changes and initiation of multiple therapies make ongoing monitoring and support from health care professionals essential to the maintenance of treatment goals.

■ The availability of multiple technology aides for improving self-management will not appeal to all patients. Balanced exposure to the benefits and burdens (including costs) of new technologies (such as CGM) will help patients make informed decisions about adoption. As with any form of intensification, variable use of technology should be assumed, with periods of suboptimal and optimal use.

- The contribution of psychological distress to glycemic status requires ongoing evaluation. Stressful lifestyles do not preclude intensive management. However, every patient should be monitored for signs of depression so that potential lack of adherence with the treatment plan can be avoided and the patient's safety assured. Potential adverse psychological consequence of intensification of treatment (e.g., depression, disordered eating behaviors, needle phobia, and the fear of hypoglycemia) should also be monitored during and after treatment. These conditions may not become evident until the patient has experienced intensive therapy and its physiological outcomes (e.g., weight gain, more frequent episodes of hypoglycemia, or the need for insulin).

- There are expected periods of psychological distress in the life course of the disease. For example, a patient's emotional response to and attitudes toward complications will interact with treatment goals to modify medical management. The presence of complications need not deter patients from attempting to improve their glucose control; however, health care providers will need to help patients modify goals of treatment if complications associated with intensive diabetes management (e.g., worsening retinopathy, weight gain, severe hypoglycemia) occur. Conversely, psychological sequelae of poor diabetes outcomes, (e.g., poor eye sight impacting lifestyle or ability to participate in certain types of physical activity) may dishearten the patient and result in loss of desire for intensive management. It is important to recognize that these reactions are normative and patients need support in adapting to functional limitations.

Psychosocial Issues

U se of intensive management during the Diabetes Control and Complications Trial (DCCT) taught us that patients can and will follow a medical regimen that is complex and multifaceted. In the period of more than 18 years since the announcement of the results of this trial, intensive diabetes management has become feasible on a wider scale, as pharmacologic therapies, advanced technologies, and increased patient awareness have increased. We also learned through the Diabetes Prevention Program (DPP) trial that, if multidisciplinary services are available, user friendly, and personalized, a high degree of compliance with a complex lifestyle-based regimen can be achieved and sustained, and there is a greater likelihood that treatment goals can be met without detrimental effects to the patient's quality of life. However, before intensification of diabetes management begins, it is important to identify which non-medical or psychosocial factors promote or interfere with a patient achieving glycemic control and how intensive management will affect the patient's quality of life and psychosocial well-being. If intensive diabetes management affects the patient's job or school performance, interpersonal relationships, and emotional well-being in a negative manner, noncompliance with the prescribed regimen is likely, as is poorer glycemic control.

ASSESSING PATIENT SUITABILITY FOR INTENSIFICATION

Many patients come to the health care provider with the stated goal of "improving my blood sugar control." However, emotional factors; lifestyle or financial barriers, and lack of, outdated, or inaccurate information may make immediate initiation of intensive management unfeasible or may suggest that the patient is unsuited to intensive treatment. Instead, patients can be offered the option of gradually intensifying self-care. Based upon a foundation of education, self-management skills that fit the patient's lifestyle and do not place an unmanageable burden on the daily routine can be added to the self-care routine one at a time.

PRACTICING BEHAVIOR

Adherence screening is recommended as a routine part of clinical practice. Adherence screening involves the following:

■ Assessment (with a questionnaire or interview format) of

- the burden on the patient of self-care tasks (What is it like to live with the required tasks on a daily basis?),
- intentions regarding self-care behavior (Does the patient intend to continue these tasks in the future?), and
- attitudes about treatment prescriptions (Does this method of treatment address the patient's goals for diabetes care?);
- screening for diabetes-related distress and depression
■ question the patient regarding whether he or she
- feels able and is willing to follow regimen changes,
- believes the changes will have a positive effect on his or her health, and
- believes the change in self-care tasks will not present an unmanageable lifestyle burden;
■ identification of gaps in the patient's knowledge, skills, and perception of self-efficacy so these issues can be addressed as part of the intervention process; and
■ allow the patient to try out and become proficient in different treatment methods and self-care behaviors.

Because there is no one right way to treat diabetes, this approach allows patients to "try on" different treatment methods without concern of failure and provides a frame of reference wherein health care providers do not label lack of success as noncompliance. Adherence screening provides the practitioner with the opportunity to assess and develop the cooperation and skills of the patient and realistically develop the "best fit" treatment regimen.

A good example of adherence screening is an approach used in the selection of patients for insulin pump use. The pump can work well for those individuals who wish to achieve glycemic control but whose daily schedule does not fit easily into a routine. The pump provides the patient with the greatest freedom of lifestyle and has been used effectively to limit weight gain in the context of glycemic control. However, the choice of the pump for insulin delivery requires greater attention to detail and compliance with self-care tasks than any other form of treatment. Therefore, asking the patient to practice the behaviors necessary for success with the insulin pump and assessing the patient's commitment to this expensive and labor-intensive treatment can save resources and prevent unnecessary frustration on the part of the patient and health care provider. Although the steps listed below are specific to the insulin pump, this approach can be translated to any form of intensified management.

■ Evaluate patient motivation and ability regarding the essential tasks associated with pump use using a multiple daily injection (MDI) routine and self-monitoring of blood glucose.
■ Assess patient facility with and psychological comfort regarding use of the pump by having the patient using a "loaner" pump.
■ Assess the patient's intention to use the pump as a long-term method of insulin delivery.
■ Assess whether the patient has the financial resources necessary for the maintenance of pump therapy; if finances prevent long-term use of this treatment method, help the patient identify acceptable therapeutic alternatives.

It is important to note that compliance is different than adherence. Compliance assumes there is an exact prescription for behavior and that the patient must fulfill all behaviors to be considered compliant. As mentioned earlier, there is "no one right way to treat diabetes." Therefore, holding a patient to "one regimen" misrepresents adherence to self-management behaviors. Systematic evaluation of adherence is unusual in clinical practice. In most cases provider evaluation of patient adherence is subjective: partially based on patient report of what they have or haven't done, substantiated, or not, by patient success in achieving glycemic control, preventing weight gain, reducing adverse events, and complications. This pre-supposes complete control of disease outcomes based on patient behaviors. Evaluation of adherence, the more appropriate term regarding diabetes self-management behaviors, requires multiple steps:

- Clear communication of expectations for self-care behaviors and expected outcomes
- A method to monitor behavior and determine efficacy
- A feedback system by which modifications to the regime can be made when necessary

PSYCHOLOGICAL STATUS AND PSYCHOSOCIAL SUPPORT SYSTEMS

Psychological distress or well-being can affect a patient's ability to carry out the behavior and communication necessary to implement and maintain intensive diabetes management. Evaluation of current and prior psychological status by a mental health professional familiar with diabetes and its care should be included with the assessment of the patient's physical status. Assessment of psychological status should predate or be ongoing during intensification.

A potential contraindication to intensification is the prior or current diagnosis of a psychiatric illness that impairs an individual's ability to carry out activities of daily living (including diabetes self-care tasks); make, evaluate, or implement treatment decisions; or maintain close contact with a provider.

If the patient is found to have impaired problem-solving abilities or judgment, and both the patient and provider wish to proceed with intensification, appropriate psychosocial supports (including treatment for the psychological issues that may affect treatment) and safeguards to monitor adverse treatment outcomes (e.g., repeated DKA or severe hypoglycemia) should be put in place as intensification of care begins.

Source(s) of motivation for intensive management are important to assess. Patient commitment to intensive management should be directly assessed by the health care provider. If motivation comes from a source outside of the individual, such as the parent of an adolescent or a spouse, the dynamics of that relationship need to be evaluated because they contribute to the success of treatment. Unless personal and family commitment to intensification is evident, diabetes management may negatively affect the patient's quality of life and/or become a vehicle for family conflict. It may become necessary to refer the patient and their support persons for further diabetes education as well as interpersonal counseling.

THE INDIVIDUAL

Intensive management, in particular, places greater burdens on the patient than do conventional treatment approaches, creating the potential for burnout, perceived failure, lowered self-esteem, and depression. The occurrence of complications that produce functional limitations, such as worsening eyesight or decreased mobility resulting from micro- and macrovascular disease, can also be sources of depression, lessening of self-esteem, and lowered quality of life. Depressive symptoms can be associated with

- diagnosis, whether the patient is being informed of increased risk or the actual development of diabetes;
- adverse effects of treatment (e.g., severe hypoglycemia, weight gain, or perceived treatment failure);
- the onset of complications;
- the negative effect of diabetes care on lifestyle or psychosocial adjustment;
- lack of real or perceived support in the home, work, school, or other social environment;
- a change in real or perceived self-image or functional abilities;
- fluctuations in physical well-being and mood associated with changes in blood glucose levels;
- increased burden, including finances, of medical care.

Patients should be monitored for signs of depression throughout the course of treatment because depression can be expected to affect motivation and the ability to carry out the prescribed self-management behaviors. Depression may be manifested by less frequent self-care behaviors or loss of interest in intensive management.

Another source of disease specific distress may be the weight gain that can occur secondary to improved control. Satisfaction with body image, particularly in adolescent and adult women, may diminish, resulting in disordered eating behaviors, including intentional insulin omission or dose reduction to lose weight through calorie wastage via glycosuria (see Eating and Body Image Disorders below).

When signs of depression are identified or disordered eating behavior is suspected, glycemic targets may need to be modified and appropriate psychosocial supports put in place to ensure the patient's safety. These supports may include, but are not limited to, initiation of individual or family psychotherapy, antidepressant medications, and hospitalization for monitoring of food intake in conjunction with insulin dose. A family member may need to be enlisted to monitor the patient's eating habits if an eating disorder is diagnosed. If counseling or psychotherapy is initiated, the effect of the patient's mood and eating patterns on self-care behaviors or, conversely, the effect of the diabetes regimen on mood and eating behavior should be evaluated and shared with the medical treatment team. The therapist/counselor can also help monitor the patient's ability to maintain self-care behaviors and assess the patient's psychosocial support system. If possible, it is important to identify sources of depressive symptomatology or subjective pressures that might lead an individual to sacrifice health or blood glucose control. The burden created by the diabetes care regimen and accountability to health care providers should be considered as potential sources of stress.

It is sometimes assumed that simply having diabetes places the patient at increased risk for psychopathology or that a patient is being noncompliant (see content above regarding adherence/compliance). When a thorough assessment is made, however, it is not uncommon to find that the source of depression, nonadherence to care regimen, or other mental health disturbance is not diabetes related. Similarly, the source of the patient's dysphoria may be external circumstance(s) that make it difficult for him or her to follow the preferred and/or prescribed regimen. Regardless of its source, depression can and often does affect care behavior. Therapists can help with treatment decisions and help family members and others (such as teachers, friends, or coworkers) learn to support needed behavior and attitude changes. When a patient is diagnosed with significant psychological problems, including the therapist in the treatment team becomes critical to the implementation and maintenance of intensive management.

ASSESSING THE EFFECT OF STRESS ON GLYCEMIC CONTROL

Stressors—positive and negative, long- or short-term—affect the individual's ability to maintain good glycemic control. The patient's response to (stress and typical level of) stress should be assessed before intensification is begun to help determine suitability for intensive treatment and to identify regimen strategies that will best maximize individual methods of coping with stress.

Transient stress causes a state of relative insulin deficiency as a result of increased concentrations of counterregulatory hormones and leads to hyperglycemia. The effects of chronic stress on glycemic control are not well understood. However, repeated sequential stress (physical or psychological) and repeated episodes of hypoglycemia alter counterregulatory responses, which may, in turn, alter the symptoms patients have comes to associate with hypoglycemia or anxiety. Changed, missing, or a blunted counterregulatory response may affect the individual's ability to identify symptoms associated with changes in blood glucose levels and those due to psychosocial stress. The identification of stress-related events and symptoms is important in identifying potential causes of high or fluctuating blood glucose levels, especially when near-normal glycemic control is the goal of treatment.

Health care practitioners can help patients who strive for glycemic control to evaluate the effects of stressful life events on blood glucose levels through the use of careful blood glucose–monitoring records in which the patient is encouraged to record life events as well as blood glucose level and insulin dose. The patient can learn how to distinguish symptoms caused by life stress, which may, in turn, affect blood glucose levels, from symptoms that might be expected from changes in blood glucose levels (e.g., feelings of hunger and light-headedness before a planned meal). Patients practicing intensive management should be encouraged to test blood glucose whenever they feel symptoms or experience psychosocial stress to identify their own pattern of glycemic response.

Although stressful lifestyles do not preclude an intensive diabetes management regimen, a patient must learn to cope effectively with changes in blood glucose levels caused by stressors and to develop and practice compensatory or substitute behaviors. Intervention strategies for stress reduction can include relaxation techniques, regular exercise regimens, support people/groups, medications, and changes in the diabetes management regimen itself. Intervention strategies should be tailored to the source of the stress, the patient's glycemic response, and the resources (psychological and other) the patient possesses to cope with the stressor. One strategy may be to

- meet with the patient and identify the source(s) of the stress,
- help the patient quantify the glycemic and emotional response to the stress,
- suggest and try out coping methods (e.g., relaxation techniques) that the patient finds acceptable,
- monitor the effectiveness of the coping strategy and its effect on blood glucose, and/or
- reevaluate the patient's subjective level of stress and make changes to coping methods as needed to improve glycemic control and emotional well-being.

Patterns of eating in response to stress also need to be addressed for individuals with both type 1 and type 2 diabetes. Patients need counseling regarding compensatory skills necessary to maintain glucose levels within the acceptable range through exercise, insulin, or medication modifications when stress-related eating is identified. Individualized long-term nutritional and psychological counseling should also be offered as an adjunct to short-term coping strategies aimed at immediate glucose control. The ultimate goal of the intervention should be a lifestyle change (in this case, eating or exercise habits) rather than an accommodation to the dysfunctional coping. The process of identification of stressors that impede maintenance of glycemic control and the development of coping strategies may best be achieved with the help of a mental health professional familiar with diabetes care who is integrated into the diabetes care team.

THE FAMILY SYSTEM

Family support is often a critical element in the success of intensive management because family members provide both concrete resources and emotional support for a patient's effort to improve his or her diabetes care. The process of intensifying treatment should be slowed and the health care provider should consider referral for counseling if a patient reports symptoms of depression related to the diabetes care regimen or if family conflict around diabetes management is manifested.

Family conflict over diabetes management can occur in any family when members disagree about treatment regimens, glycemic goals, and burdens of care. Families who are particularly susceptible are those with

- a teenage patient whose bid for autonomy and independence from parental caretaking results in worsening control;
- young children, when responsibility for care is unequal between parents (parents do not share health concerns such as what to glycemic targets are not achieved or the long-term consequences of poor glycemic control);
- a perception that the diabetes care routine negatively affects the family environment (regardless of the age of the patient);
- experience with poor control that results in repeated episodes of severe hypoglycemia or diabetic ketoacidosis, necessitating frequent hospitalizations or trips to the emergency room (conversely, family conflict may precipitate these episodes); and/or

■ psychosocial and material resources disproportionately expended on the family member with diabetes, making other family members feel that their needs are not being met (this applies to spouses as well as siblings).

It is particularly important for the practitioner to assess the family system regarding attitudes toward intensification and medical care in general, willingness to participate in diabetes care, and financial resources. Conflicts can be avoided by making a clear diabetes care contract with all participating family members that specifies who will take responsibility for which aspects of the regimen, the monitoring functions of each family member, and how the care regimen will or won't affect how the family lives. If a patient who wants intensification lives alone, identify appropriate support people who will commit to regular contact with the individual and be willing to assume responsibility for monitoring the well-being of the patient, especially with regard to adverse events such as severe hypoglycemia.

Parents are increasingly seeking intensive treatment for their young children and adolescents with type 1 diabetes and are initiating prevention efforts on behalf of their overweight children or adolescents who have pre-diabetes. Long-term concerns about the physical well-being of their child place an enormous burden on many parents. Thus, parents may have desires for an intensive treatment regimen that may not be feasible given the age and maturity of the child or goals that are not shared by the child or adolescent or stress the family system beyond functionality. Issues of autonomy and decision making regarding adherence to the prescribed treatment regimen can lead to family conflict, regardless of the age of the patient. Decisions about the treatment regimen should be considered in the context of the desires, adjustment to illness, resources, and abilities of all members who constitute the family system, especially when formulating regimens for children and adolescents. These caveats also apply to spousal systems and adult children taking care of elderly parents with diabetes. Imposition of a lifestyle tailored to intensive diabetes management may place restrictions on the routines and food environment in the home and requires taking responsibility for maintaining the regimen that affects all members of the household. It may be particularly difficult to motivate an adolescent with pre-diabetes to make lifestyle changes or even to consider him- or herself as having a disease when he or she does not experience symptoms and/or is not required to take medication for the condition.

ASSESSING COPING SKILLS

ASSESSMENT OF DIABETES-RELATED COPING

Effective diabetes-related coping involves

■ identifying those factors contributing to current and near-future glycemic status (e.g., life stress, change in routine, physical stress or comorbidities, caloric intake, exercise, alcohol or medication use, insulin dose, and pump failure),

- having the knowledge and skills to evaluate the circumstances and respond appropriately.
- implementing a new treatment strategy or behavior.
- having access and willingness to use a health care professional or support person who can help solve problems and collaborate in a treatment decision.

Coping skills can be taught and practiced. Coping skills involve making prompt and effective changes to the diabetes care regimen when a problem arises. However, assessment of the patient's willingness to take responsibility for treatment decisions or to use a support person to aid in decision making can help avoid adverse events (e.g., severe hypoglycemia or ketoacidosis caused by over- or undertreatment of glucose levels, a foot sore that becomes a bone lesion because the patient ignored it rather than seeking prompt treatment).

The patient's ability to cope with life events unrelated to having diabetes should be monitored, along with his or her ability to cope with the requirements of intensive management. During routine management visits, the patient's willingness to assume responsibility for regimen changes should be reevaluated. Communication between patient and care provider prevents burnout caused by the intensive diabetes regimen, as well as patient–provider misunderstandings regarding responsibility for care. Many patients are willing to let decision making rest with their health care providers, seeking guidance when they are unsure or unwilling to take responsibility for treatment decisions. Although this is an acceptable practice pattern, the "contract" between the patient and the caregiver must be explicit.

If a pattern of trusting communication has been established between the patient and caregivers, diabetes-related coping strategies can be tried by the patient in the context of the safety net provided by the support system. Once the patient is fully competent and able to solve problems related to his or her glucose control, the "contract" for decision making and taking responsibility should be renegotiated. Increased practice with diabetes-related problem solving and effective self-care behaviors will increase the patient's ability to cope with the effects of stressful life events. However, the support of health care providers is essential to the patients' sense of well-being. Effective self-care behavior achieved through patient–provider communication will contribute to overall glycemic control and feelings of diabetes-related self-confidence, efficacy, and well-being.

Use of technologic aides such as direct uploading doses and blood sugar values from a pump can facilitate this communication. Further, electronic media such as email and Twitter can replace phone calls or face-to-face meetings, allowing both patient and provider flexibility and ease of contact. As with other recommendations for care, it is important to establish which channels will be used and frequency of communication so that expectations are clear between providers and patients. It is also important that a clear understanding be developed between patient, support personnel, and care providers regarding issues of privacy and who will be privy to this information, particularly if underage children/adolescents are involved or there are concerns for safety.

Intensification of treatment, as well as adoption of adherence aids, may involve public exposure of the patient's disease condition. Behaviors may be required throughout the day when the patient cannot retire to a private location to, for example, test blood glucose or give an insulin bolus. Thus, intensification may also involve patients' coming to terms with the expectations and beliefs of others, becoming a patient advocate and educator. This may or may not feel comfortable to the individual and, as with other coping behaviors, the issue of private vs public "business" may need to be addressed and practiced. It is a common experience for with diabetes to be asked, "Are you supposed to be eating that" or, even more pointedly, told they are not supposed to be eating food with sugar. Having planned responses to welcome or unwelcome "misguided helping" is part of living with diabetes. Anticipating such interactions are part of basic diabetes education, but may need revisiting during the process of intensification.

IDENTIFYING PSYCHOSOCIAL RESOURCES

Interpersonal support, or lack thereof, often contributes significantly to a patient's ability to implement and maintain intensive management. Psychosocial support can help remove barriers to adherence because it eases the burden of illness.

Support can come from a variety of sources: the health care team, a specific provider, a family member, a religious organization, or a diabetes support group. The support offered can assume a variety of forms:

- emotional support that affirms patients' desires to intensify their diabetes care and improve their health;
- endoresement of treatment decisions;
- a safety net to cope with adverse events;
- a source of resources (e.g., financial aid provided when health care providers identify rebate programs from pharmaceutical companies or put patients in touch with discount supply companies); and
- care provider (physician, nurse, educator, CDE) help with self-care behaviors.

A patient's need for support varies in the same manner that an individual's response to stress varies. Most patients need education about available resources. Management visits can be used to help identify psychosocial resources in the patient's community and in the medical community. Patients will be most comfortable seeking support from those people with whom and institutions with which they have established relationships and feel most trusting. Therefore, continuity of care providers becomes an essential part of intensive management. Although patients may be familiar with support groups, they may not realize that educational programs and regional support groups are routinely available and that hospitals in the community may offer diabetes care specialty teams. The health care practitioner can

- ask patients to identify individuals in their lives who would be willing to be educated to help with intensive diabetes management,
- include significant others in the planning of diabetes care regimens,

- encourage patients to share the responsibilities of diabetes care with family and friends to whatever extent they feel comfortable, and
- stress that intensive management of diabetes brings the increased risk of severe hypoglycemia and involving others in diabetes care can provide safeguards against this risk.

SUPPORTING AND MAINTAINING PATIENTS' BEHAVIOR CHANGES

Patient motivation, ability, and intention to maintain a complex regimen will vary over time. Choosing to focus less on on diabetes care during periods of emotional turmoil, holidays, and vacation is to be expected. Other life events may temporarily take precedence over intensive diabetes management. Understanding that variation in self-management behaviors is expected (not aberrant), the practitioner can approach problem solving without a sense of failure and frustration with the patient. Attempt to determine why the lapse in self-care behavior occurred, and enlist the patient in making decisions regarding the redirection of treatment. Redirection and refocusing by the health care team should be conferred in a collaborative, nonjudgmental manner.

Intensification of diabetes management requires the patient to prioritize the diabetes care regimen. Health care providers should enlist all possible supports for their patients to lessen the burden of treatment.

- Ongoing education and training in skill acquisition, including diabetes-related problem solving, are necessary components of intensive management.
- Treatment goals should be defined, monitored, and redefined as patients successfully master each skill and reach benchmarks in care.
- Find those strategies that fit lifestyle needs.
- Lapses in self-care behaviors should be expected as a routine part of care and do not constitute treatment failure.

Ongoing adherence with the diet and exercise prescriptions are the most difficult aspects of care for many patients, regardless of other therapeutic modalities. Like other areas targeted for behavior change, diet and exercise require ongoing long-term monitoring and modification of treatment goals according to the patient's success with the intervention strategy. Interpersonal support is particularly useful when changing lifestyle habits such as diet and exercise. The presence of a fitness instructor on the team or access to a gym that offers classes can make the difference between maintaining exercise regimens or returning to a baseline, inactive lifestyle. Active monitoring by a nutritionist can reinforce new eating patterns and helps the patient make the connection between better nutrition and improved glycemic control. The connection between new behaviors and glycemic control may not be immediate. Positive regard for small steps in behavior change may provide the support necessary until the patient's behavior becomes self-sustaining (see Lifestyle Changes later in this chapter).

Helping patients formulate a regimen that is responsive to their lifestyles will help ensure greater compliance with the prescribed treatment. A treatment regimen that fits into, rather than controls, lifestyle should be the goal of an attainable treatment plan. Patients can be instructed on self-care behaviors and strategies to improve glycemic status that take into account current glucose value, planned physical activity, and planned caloric intake. When a patient is resistant to a health care provider's suggestions, noncompliance should not be assumed. A collaborative dialogue between patient and provider can reestablish a working plan about self-management wherein the patient agrees to glycemic goals and together strategies are developed that work toward resumption of tight control.

ADOPTION OF NEW THERAPIES AND THERAPEUTIC MODALITIES

The advent of oral agents that increase insulin sensitivity and glucose metabolism, or inhibit carbohydrate metabolism, or hormonal analogues such as pramlintide, which changes gastric emptying and satiety, have added new treatment options to intensive management strategies. In addition, new technological advances such as "smart" pumps and continuous glucose monitoring with subcutaneous glucose sensors have changed the manner and intensity of treatment. Adoption of these technologies requires achieving a balance between the potential for fine-tuning glycemia and retaining an acceptable quality of life. Not all patients will eagerly embrace the ability to frequently monitor blood glucose levels, no matter how easy, in order to make changes in insulin dosing. Not all patients will elect to give themselves an additional pre-meal injection of pramlintide. Selecting which new agents and technologies to incorporate into the regimen should be negotiated in the same manner that other aspects of the regimen are modified. When educating patients about newer oral agents (including thiazolidinediones, metformin, orlistat, and acarbose, DPP-IV inhibitors) and injected agents (such as pramlintide and exenatide), caregivers should be clear in communicating which medications are used as adjunctive therapies, which are primary therapies for glucose control, and which have novel effects that differ from their current medications.

Caution is urged regarding suggesting that insulin can be eliminated if patients are willing to agree to a multi-therapy oral regimen. As of this writing, it is not definitively known whether the same level of glycemic control can be achieved for most patients using multiple oral therapies vs insulin plus oral therapy. Therefore, promising a patient that insulin will not be used could be misleading or a set up for feeling as if the patient failed treatment should there be a clear need to begin insulin use. Most patients with type 2 diabetes will ultimately benefit from insulin, so this option should be presented to the patient as an acceptable alternative to achieve good glycemic control rather than a perceived punishment for failure.

Goals for treatment should be realistic and attainable. For example, a 350-lb (159-kg) patient with type 2 diabetes might benefit from adjunctive therapy with acarbose and orlistat. However, discontinuing insulin might not be an attainable goal until major weight loss occurs. Some drugs may require frequent monitoring of liver function, requiring more office visits. If the benefit-to-cost ratio is clearly explained to the patient, better compliance is likely.

New pharmacologic agents; new technologies for assessing blood glucose, ketone, and glycated hemoglobin (A1c) values; new methods of insulin administration; and the personnel whose job is to promote and encourage patient success have greatly enhanced patients' abilities to achieve glycemic control. However, health care providers need to be aware that "one size doesn't fit all" in diabetes treatment when considering use of the entire treatment armamentarium for our patients. In particular, carefully consider age and cognitive abilities, as well as emotional, financial, and health care resources, on an individual basis when introducing multiple therapies into the diabetes care regimen. Adoptive of intensive regimen strategies and technologies are best presented as enhancements to care that can be variably and variously used to problem solve as well as help attain glycemic goals. Care should be taken not to present adjunctive therapies as punishment for treatment failure.

For example, if a single mother requests intensification of treatment for her type 1 diabetes without adequate health care coverage, recommending self-monitoring of blood glucose five times per day may present financial as well as lifestyle difficulties. However, her desire to remain healthy for the wellbeing of her children may provide motivation to intensify her regimen. An MDI regimen plus access to online pharmaceutical sources could potentially overcome barriers presented by her financial constraints and lifestyle. In a similar vein, older but "healthy" individual with diabetes may experience the demands of intensification as overwhelming simply because they represent so much change in the patients' usual daily routine or stressful if the patient cannot access the necessary resources. Conversely, an older adult may seek intensification and use of multiple therapies and technologies because they now have more time and resources to devote to diabetes care, and seek to improve their health status. Patients should be encouraged to realistically assess whether, with support, they can implement and incorporate all the regimen behaviors that we ask of them. Accepting modified treatment goals and gradual implementation of different therapeutic tools, with the aim of achieving the best glucose control possible, is suggested to prevent burnout in patients and practitioners.

HELPING PATIENTS WITH LONG-TERM ADHERENCE

The suggestion to initiate intensive management of diabetes may come from the patient, friend or family of the patient, or the provider. However, if patient and provider do not agree on the methods and goals of treatment, if the appropriate education and resources are not provided or available, or if the patient is unable (for whatever functional or practical reason) to carry out the treatment tasks, then treatment "failure" will probably occur. Health care providers traditionally have attributed treatment failure to noncompliance on the part of the patient. We now know that poor adherence may be the result of a number of factors in addition to treatment complexity, including

- barriers to adherence, such as lack of resources or access to care;
- lack of clarity and/or poor communication of expected behaviors or regimen prescription;
- lack of patient motivation or efficacy; and/or
- patient non-participation in the treatment contract.

Patients are often afraid to tell their health care providers that they feel incapable of carrying out the requested behavior, are disinclined because of fear or lack of resources, or disagree with the regimen prescription in the first place. A patient's willingness to use the education and resources provided by caregivers is crucial to the implementation of intensive management. Patients who do not feel rapport with their caregivers are less likely to incorporate and sustain changes to their care regimen. A patient's willingness to use the resources provided by caregivers also is necessary to help prevent adverse events secondary to the treatment, such as severe hypoglycemia or transient worsening of eyesight. Establishing an atmosphere of collaboration and mutual respect will help to obtain the patient's cooperation with regard to carrying out the treatment plan and following the advice given by the provider. It is important to

- include patients and their support network in the treatment team;
- define and agree on treatment goals and the self-care behaviors that are required to achieve and maintain these goals;
- adapt the regimen to the patient's lifestyle;
- include the patient in regimen choice;
- provide the necessary education, support, and training for skill acquisition of self-care behaviors;
- have patients practice self-care behaviors;
- monitor the efficacy and outcomes of the behaviors that have been agreed to;
- monitor and redefine goals as necessary;
- renegotiate the care plan or behaviors if the current plan has not been successful;
- make incremental changes;
- expect periods of lessened adherence; and
- expect periods of poor performance and uneven glycemic results as patients learn new skills or their life circumstances change.

Above all, it is crucial to not automatically assume noncompliance with the treatment regimen when facing treatment failure.

Note that treatment behaviors that have been mutually agreed on may not always result in the expected glycemic outcome. Factors such as stress reactivity, other disease processes, or changes in lifestyle or routine may result in unanticipated regimen effects. Caregivers and patients engaged in achieving glycemic control should not view unanticipated outcomes as failures of treatment. Instead, patient and caregiver can work to identify causal relationships between lifestyle, emotion, and glycemic status to develop self-care coping strategies. For example, stress produced by school- or job-related responsibilities can cause a rise in blood glucose. The individual may have completed self-care tasks as prescribed and may have attempted to compensate for anticipated stress by extra blood tests, extra insulin, and/or less food. These strategies may not have the anticipated effect on blood glucose or may produce an effect later in the day. The response can be documented and used to decide future strategies. Help the patient understand that unexpected glycemic excursions should not be viewed as a personal failure, poor problem solving, or treatment failure.

LIFESTYLE CHANGES

Weight management and exercise are two treatment strategies traditionally prescribed for all patients with diabetes that have, because of their inherent difficulties, taken a back seat to pharmacological therapies. The significant contribution of weight loss and daily physical activity to glucose metabolism, as well as to quality of life, overall health, and the sense of well-being, is increasingly emphasized in diabetes management. As weight-related diabetes and associated cardiovascular risk continues to increase in all segments of the population, basic lifestyle behaviors have increasingly been the target of interventions.

Results of the Diabetes Prevention Program (DPP) and United Kingdom Prospective Diabetes Study (UKPDS) have shown us that lifestyle changes, particularly diet and exercise modification, must be implemented in addition to intensification of self-care behaviors to achieve optimal metabolic control. As a result, the role of health care practitioners has expanded to include helping patients initiate and maintain lifestyle changes that support intensive diabetes management. Health care providers, with the exception of behaviorists, often express that they are not equipped for this role, citing lack of training in behavioral interventions, lack of time, and poor reimbursement for these services. Although use of a multidisciplinary team to support patients is optimal, the practitioner is often expected to initiate and/or monitor diet and exercise interventions in addition to the traditional medical management of the patient. Strategies are needed to achieve these goals within a primary care setting.

Cognitive behavioral therapy within a context of social support has been shown to be effective in increasing exercise and modifying dietary intake, resulting in weight loss and improved glycemic control and cardiac risk factors. The same techniques have been applied to intensification of self-care behaviors. Behavior modification is a multistep process that includes

- establishing a set of beliefs regarding the efficacy of the new behavior (education),
- learning the new behavior (skill building),
- practicing the new behavior (rehearsal),
- overcoming barriers to implementation of the behavior (problem solving), and
- preventing recidivism to the old behavior pattern by monitoring well-being and adverse events associated with lapses in treatment (relapse prevention).

Targeting and monitoring a single behavior change until that skill is mastered and integrated into the patient's lifestyle makes this process manageable and easily incorporated into a routine diabetes care visit. For example, 30–60 minutes of moderate to vigorous activity at least five times a week, intake of five to nine fruits and vegetables per day, and caloric intake that matches energy expenditure is recommended to prevent weight gain during intensification of glucose control. These goals can be overwhelming and seem unattainable to the patient if presented as a packaged prescription for good health. Entering into a "contract" with the patient and agreeing to smaller, more manageable goals in a stepwise fashion enhances the likelihood of success. The following are steps to a contracting process.

- Educate the patient regarding self-management behavior necessary to achieve good glycemic control.
- Identify a behavior that the patient is willing to work to change (e.g., ask "Would you be willing to walk a half hour daily or eat two servings of vegetables daily?"), not one that is "prescribed."
- Define the behavior in such a way that change can be monitored (e.g., have the patients keep a daily activity log noting the type of activity, time, and duration; keep a food record only for lunch each day).
- Set a realistic goal for the change that you and the patient agree on (e.g., increase walking from zero times a week to three times a week for a half hour, *not* increase exercise from zero times a week to running three miles three times a week).
- Establish and agree on the methods and supports necessary for the patient to change his or her daily routine (e.g., "What time of day would be convenient for this particular activity?").
- Set a realistic date to accomplish the goal and for discussing the progress the patient has made using his or her written record.
- If a routine checkup is not scheduled, arrange to communicate with the patient after about 2 weeks about his or her progress, successes, and setbacks, during which time it is important to identify barriers to success, generate problem-solving solutions, or modify the goal to make it either more manageable or challenging.
- At the appointed follow-up visit or through electronic media, assess with the patient whether the new behavior has been mastered or more time is needed to make the behavior routine. If life circumstances have changed, more problem solving may be needed, along with another plan for ensuring maintenance of the new behavior.

The practitioner may choose to develop a document that contains these key elements, which is filled out and agreed to during the "consultation" that follows the physical examination. Preliminary discussion of the behavior to be targeted and the goal to be achieved can occur while the examination takes place. This allows patients time to reflect on whether they are motivated to tackle changing a particular behavior at this particular time, consider whether the behavior is realistic for them, and they can develop a feasible plan to implement the change. Presenting alternative behavior strategies can help the patient make realistic choices and not feel afraid of "disappointing" the care provider. It is helpful to introduce discussion of the patient's social support system at this time.

Lifestyle change is easier to accomplish if social supports are in place. For example, if a wife is willing to walk with her spouse for 45 minutes each day before dinner and the husband agrees to this partnership, there is a greater likelihood that the exercise will occur. Similarly, if a spouse doesn't mind that only no-calorie sodas are available at home, the patient will have an easier time reducing caloric intake. When opportunities to exercise are available and are not disruptive to the family routine, the individual is more likely to maintain the exercise pattern. Incorporating significant others into the behavior change—whether it be in dietary pattern, exercise, or self-care behaviors—lightens the burden on the patient through sharing of responsibility and implicit social support. Conversely, if discussion of social supports makes apparent existing conflicts with family members regarding implementation of lifestyle changes, bringing significant others to follow-up visits is indicated for education and problem solving.

Once a contract is agreed to and documented (including significant others when appropriate), the practitioner or designated office personnel can follow up by phone, fax, email, or in person to monitor the "intervention." Again, if patients are counseled that setbacks and difficulties are expected when changing lifestyle behaviors, a sense of failure can be attenuated if not prevented. Often, small changes in behavior not only improve the patient's medical outcome but improve quality of life and enhance his or her feelings of efficacy and well-being.

Behavior management techniques that address lifestyle needs and the monitoring of regimen behaviors, including nutrition and exercise, can be incorporated into the diabetes care plan under the supervision of a

- psychologist–certified diabetes educator (CDE),
- nutritionist–CDE with behavioral training,
- diabetes nurse educator who is already monitoring blood glucose as well as other lifestyle behaviors, and
- fitness instructor who is familiar with nutrition and diabetes management

Incorporating and monitoring efforts at weight management and fitness are accepted standards of care for all people with diabetes. When implementing these therapies, it is essential that appropriate professional personnel are identified to initiate, monitor, and motivate patient goal setting.

POTENTIAL ADVERSE PSYCHOLOGICAL OUTCOMES OF TREATMENT

DEPRESSION

There is ample evidence that patients with diabetes have a higher than expected prevalence of depressive disorders. The relationship between depression and diabetes appears to be bidirectional such that each may contribute to the other. Depression in individuals with diabetes has been implicated in noncompliance with self-care behaviors, lack of motivation to intensify treatment, poorer quality of life, and worsened glycemic control. It is believed that depression is underdiagnosed in this population; however, it should not automatically be assumed that all nonadherence, lack of motivation for intensive management, and suboptimal quality of life are the result of depressive symptomatology. Thus, depression screening should be an integral and ongoing part of intensive diabetes management. The easiest and most direct method to achieve this goal of treatment is to administer a short, standardized depression-screening instrument that asks about changes in mood, level of interest in usual activities (including diabetes care), food intake, sleep patterns, relationships, and any changes in functional ability (e.g., ability to maintain job function, keep up with school tasks or diabetes care tasks). If screening identifies problems in any of these areas, further evaluation by a qualified mental health professional is indicated.

EATING AND BODY IMAGE DISORDERS

Disordered eating behavior is commonly reported among patients with both-type 1 and type 2 diabetes. Treatment prescriptions such as restrained eating, strict monitoring of food intake, and use of insulin (which potentiates hunger) are thought to create a fertile environment for the development of disordered eating behavior, especially because good glycemic control is often associated with weight gain. Many individuals inadvertently or purposely attempt weight stabilization via glycosuria (less than optimal glucose control) after intensive diabetes management is initiated. An eating disorder must be considered when patients routinely manipulate insulin or purge to rid themselves of calories while maintaining acceptable A1c levels and body weight. Patients who suffer from eating disorders are placing themselves at increased risk when tightening their glycemic control, in that manipulation of either calories or insulin or falsification of records to hide elevated blood glucose levels further increases the risk of hypoglycemia and/or diabetic ketoacidosis. Furthermore, disordered eating behavior has been associated with an increased rate of complications such as retinopathy and neuropathy.

Glucose control is inextricably linked to the prescription of controlled eating and the potential to gain weight. An internal conflict may occur wherein food becomes the gateway to physical health and to a loss of control over one's appearance. Gaining weight may result in resistance to adhering to the prescribed insulin regimen, severe calorie restriction, preoccupation with exercise, or other behaviors associated with aberrant eating patterns. This internal conflict—good health versus loss of control over weight (body image)—can result in a variety of subclinical and clinically diagnosable eating and body image disorders. Preliminary evidence suggests that if a patient is experiencing dysphoria and weight/body dissatisfaction, they are more likely to adopt disordered eating behaviors.

Fortunately, the prevalence of diagnosable disorders is low. However, intensification of diabetes management can further increase the risk. Subclinical dysphoria and weight-related distress are often overlooked because the patient does not want to bring attention to either aberrant eating behaviors or noncompliance with a regimen prescription such as underdosing of insulin. Unless cued by the patient, the practitioner may not ask questions that specifically address these issues. Early intervention can often prevent the development of a full-blown eating disorder, thus creating an atmosphere wherein weight concers become a part of treatment.

Discussion with patient of the likelihood of gaining weight and the stress of increased attention to food should begin as soon as the topic of intensive treatment is broached. Asking about satisfaction with weight and body size provides a starting point to integrate healthy weight management strategies into the treatment regimen. When intensification brings weight gain, evaluation of weight concerns should begin: Is the patient distressed by the weight gain associated with improving glycemic control? Is the provider concerned because the patient's weight status is putting them at risk for other diseases? Although women have a higher incidence of disordered eating behaviors, societal focus on the thinness ideal may be contributing to sub-clinical eating and body image disorders that can go undetected in both men and women. Weight concerns are no longer gender specific. Family attitudes about weight and size should also be assessed, in order to evaluate whether added pressure is being placed on the patient. Including weight management as an outcome of treatment also makes the topic a legitimate area of monitoring and concern for the patient, rather than the health care provider and patient categorizing such concerns as dysfunctional. If necessary, the services of a mental health professional can be introduced to the patient's care.

FEAR OF HYPOGLYCEMIA

Another common area of psychosocial distress associated with intensive treatment is fear of hypoglycemia. More frequent episodes of hypoglycemia can be expected when blood glucose levels hover around the normal range, the goal of intensive management. Individuals vary significantly regarding their risk and adaptive behavior, their ability to recognize hypoglycemia symptoms, and the social support they receive for monitoring and recognizing episodes of hypoglycemia. Physiologic factors (usual level of blood glucose, length of illness, and presence of complications) plays an important role in the patient's ability to recognize his or her symptoms, and the overlap between symptoms of hypoglycemia and anxiety can make recognition of episodes difficult.

Patients learn to fear hypoglycemia not only for the potential adverse physical outcomes, but also for the lack of control that results from neuroglycopenia (low blood glucose in the brain). Patients experiencing hypoglycemia may act silly, risqué, angry, or irresponsible; take risks; or withdraw. Altered personality characteristics are common. Low blood glucose levels can affect interactions with partners and coworkers, cause mistakes in mental processing, or alter physical functioning (e.g., cause automobile accidents), all of which are beyond the control of the patient during a hypoglycemic episode. As a result, patients should be concerned about excessive and/or severe hypoglycemia and should learn to take appropriate steps to avoid hypoglycemia. Some patients, however, develop a maladaptive fear of hypoglycemia that leads them to actively avoid near-normoglycemia, which is counterproductive to intensive management.

Fear of hypoglycemia should be suspected if a patient's blood glucose levels gradually or abruptly rise following an episode of hypoglycemia, for no discernible reason, or if the patient is inappropriately eliminating or excessively reducing insulin doses in relation to blood glucose levels after a period of repeated or severe hypoglycemia. Counseling about the likelihood of increased episodes of hypoglycemia and compensatory monitoring of blood glucose levels should also precede intensification, but fear of hypoglycemia should be addressed whenever it is suspected. Teach strategies to increase recognition of symptoms, prevent low blood glucose by temporarily reducing insulin doses, or increase the frequency of blood glucose monitoring (e.g., before and after exercise, before driving), along with the other skills necessary for intensive management. As above, though training those in their home or work environment to recognize and treat hypoglycemia/severe hypoglycemia is usually part of basic diabetes education, this issue should be revisited as part of intensification. This can be a forum that allows the patient to express their prior experiences and concerns about public disclosure of their disease, treatment, and consequences. If fear of hypoglycemia becomes an impediment to achieving glucose control, consider referring the patient to a mental health professional who specializes in diabetes.

NEEDLE PHOBIA

Many individuals who must use insulin initially express fear of taking injections but quickly accommodate, out of necessity, to giving themselves shots. In most cases, firm expectations for the patient's behavior (along with social support and skill building) effectively reduce fear and anxiety. When anxiety and avoidant behavior increase around giving injections, needle phobia may be operating. Avoidant behaviors can include, but are not limited to, rituals that prolong the period before the shot is given, intense expressions of distress (moaning, crying, yelling) accompanied by physical withdrawal from the needle, or frank refusal to take shots.

When needle phobia is suspected, an evaluation by a qualified mental health professional is indicated. Cognitive behavioral therapy, relaxation techniques, and other forms of psychotherapy and pharmacotherapy are effective in reducing phobic behavior and accompanying anxiety. Insulin pump therapy can also be considered, although pump malfunctions will require the use of occasional injections. The "pump solution" (often suggested by parents to reduce the distress of their child) will not solve the problem. Regardless of the intervention strategies used, it is important that the patient receive pragmatic and nonjudgmental messages about the necessity of overcoming his or her fears. At the same time, acknowledge the degree of distress that the patient is experiencing so that appropriate psychological treatment can occur. Even if the patient begins pump therapy, continue behavioral intervention to reduce anxiety associated with shot giving.

Include significant others in the intervention strategy because the patient's dysfunctional coping may be inadvertently supported, encouraged, and maintained within the context of family dynamics. A prime example of this is a mother who, when the child is diagnosed, grimaces and cries every time her child receives an injection. The child learns to associate negative emotions and distress with receiving a shot even though there may be little physical pain. When the child shows distress at shot time and shot-giving time is prolonged, especially when the parent expresses that they are "hurting" the child, the message to the child is that injections are to be avoided. In these circumstances, needle phobia may evolve: Not only does the child avoid a "painful distressing stimulus," but he or she also receives nurturing and support for the avoidant behavior. In a situation such as this, include both mother and child in the intervention.

Patients may also arrive at the point of requiring insulin with a preexisting fear of injections that intensifies when they are faced with a lifetime of self-injection. Helping patients understand the source of their fear and providing coping strategies that enable patients to successfully implement their diabetes care behaviors may reduce anxiety. In the situation where a patient with type 2 diabetes must begin using insulin, the patient may perceive that he or she has "failed" treatment. Rather than view injections as a constant reminder of this failure, help the patient understand that injections are a powerful tool to achieve glycemic control. Earlier initiation of insulin use during the course of treatment for type 2 diabetes may also prevent patients from feeling that they are being "punished" for being a "bad" (i.e., noncompliant) patient.

HELPING PATIENTS DEAL WITH COMPLICATIONS

Much of what patients believe about the inevitability of complications associated with diabetes is based on the experience of others they know with diabetes and diabetes "folklore." Treatment of diabetes has changed significantly in the past 15–20 years that many patients do not know that good control can prevent or reduce the occurrence of complications. As shown by the DCCT and the United Kingdom Prospective Diabetes Study (UKPDS), serious complications (e.g., blindness, amputations) are no longer inevitable outcomes of diabetes. However, many patients continue to believe that a downward physical spiral is unavoidable and express feelings of helplessness with regard to altering the course of their illness. If patients' attempts to achieve desired glycemic targets have not succeeded, then negative attitudes, such as those regarding their control over the development of complications, may be reinforced. These attitudes should be addressed as part of the intensification process. Successful experience with intensive regimen behaviors, such as adjustment of insulin doses in response to current glycemia, can change patient attitudes about the efficacy of the treatment. Success with short-term goals can help alter patient attitudes about the inevitability of complications and bolster intentions to continue intensive management.

Complications can exact a psychological toll and may affect a patient's ability to carry out intensive management. Physical limitations or the inability to recognize hypoglycemia secondary to complications should be directly discussed with the patient. When a complication such as gastroparesis requires a change in the treatment plan, the treatment team can expect the need for a period of transition in patient attitude and behavior. It can be anticipated that transient depression might interrupt patient adherence to prescribed regimen behaviors and necessitate appropriate team support. Care providers need to understand that dysphoria in response to the diagnosis of complications is an expected and normal response.

Patients often begin to see themselves as handicapped or limited in their ability to carry out an intensive diabetes care regimen once complications are diagnosed. Perceived limitations may be physical or emotional. In particular, complications that are related to symptom recognition, such as blunted catecholamine response or autonomic neuropathy, directly affect the patient's ability to recognize hypoglycemia. Gastroparesis significantly impacts caloric intake and thus glycemic control. Onset of these and other complications may be associated with a decline in optimism about treatment efficacy, resulting in less motivation to intensify efforts and reduced quality of well-being. Education regarding different treatment approaches and supports can help renew the patient's commitment to achieving better glycemic control. Patients may need help understanding that any improvement in their glycemic status can improve their overall health status and help retard the onset and progression of complications.

Patients should be educated about the known potential complications of treatment at the outset of intensification, so that potential worsening of physical status can be anticipated and appropriate emotional and regimen support can be provided during transition periods. Strategies to avoid potential complications should be explored and, when possible, the treatment plan should incorporate strategies to minimize these complications. Adverse events commonly associated with intensive management are

- weight gain (see Chapter 9, Nutrition Management),
- severe hypoglycemia (see Chapter 8, Monitoring), and
- transient worsening of diabetic retinopathy
- hypoglycemia unawareness (see Chapter 8, Monitoring).

These adverse outcomes may result in intentional worsening of control on the part of the patient. Patients need to develop regimen strategies and emotional supports to cope with these possibilities and maintain a long-term perspective.

CONCLUSION

Intensive management offers the patient flexibility of lifestyle and the opportunity to enhance the quality of diabetes-related life and general well-being. The importance of psychosocial and medical supports in facilitating the implementation and maintenance of intensive diabetes management should not be underestimated. The availability of multidisciplinary services and support can relieve the patient and the family of some of the burden of diabetes care. Through the incorporation of the patient and the psychosocial support system into the care team, individualized lifestyle-based regimens can be formulated, self-care behaviors can be practiced, and treatment goals can be chosen and monitored. Each patient will require an individualized treatment regimen and a unique constellation of support services, depending on age, social circumstances, psychological status, and financial resources.

Some patients are not appropriate candidates for complex intensive treatment regimens. However, diabetes management with the goal of achieving near-normal blood glucose levels can be implemented incrementally, and glycemic targets can be modified based on ongoing monitoring of treatment efficacy. The practice of intensive management of diabetes requires the commitment and dedication of patients, their unique support systems, and the health care team on an ongoing, long-term basis.

BIBLIOGRAPHY

American Diabetes Association: Standards of medical care in Diabetes. (Position Statement). *Diabetes Care* 35 (Suppl. 1):S11–S63, 2012

Anderson RJ, Freedland KE, Clouse RE, Lustman PJ: The prevalence of comorbid depression in adults with diabetes: a meta-analysis. *Diabetes Care* 24 (6):1069–1078, 2001

Diabetes Control and Complications Trial Research Group: The effect of intensive treatment of diabetes on the development and progression of long-term complications in insulin-dependent diabetes mellitus. *The New England Journal of Medicine* 329:977–986, 1993

Diabetes Control and Complications Trial Research Group: Implementation of treatment protocols in the Diabetes Control and Complications Trial. *Diabetes Care* 18:361–376, 1995

Diabetes Research in Children Network (DirecNet) Study Group. Psychological aspects of continuous glucose monitoring in pediatric type 1 diabetes. *Pediatr Diabetes* 7:32-8, 2006

DPP Research Group: The Diabetes Prevention Program (DPP): Description of lifestyle intervention. *Diabetes Care* 25:2165-2171, 2002

Eaton WW, Armenian H, Gallo J, et al: Depression and risk for onset of type II diabetes. A prospective population-based study. *Diabetes Care* 19 (10):1097–1102, 1996

Egede LE, Osborn CY: Role of motivation in the relationship between depression, self-care, and glycemic control in adults with type 2 diabetes. *The Diabetes Educator* 36:276–283, 2010

Fisher L, Glasgow RE, Strycker LA: The relationship between diabetes distress and clinical depression with glycemic control amoung patients with type 2 diabetes. *Diabetes Care* 33:1034-1036, 2010

Harkness E, Macdonald W, Valderas J, Coventry P, Gask L, Bower P: Identifying psychosocial interventions that improve both physical and mental health in patients with diabetes: A systematic review and meta-analysis. *Diabetes Care* 33:926-930, 2010

Herpertz S, Wagener R, Albus C, Kocnar M, Wagner R, Best F, Schleppinghoff BS, Filz H-P, Foerster K, Thomas W, Mann K, Koehle K, Senf W: Diabetes mellitus and eating disorders: a multicenter study on the comorbidity of the two diseases. *J Psychosomatic Res* 44(3–4):503–515, 1998

Hummer K, Vannatta J, Thompson D: Locus of control and metabolic control of diabetes: A meta-analysis. *The Diabetes Educator* 37:104–110, 2011

Karlson B, Agardh CD: Burden of illness, metabolic control, and complications in relation to depressive symptoms in IDDM patients. *Diabet Med* 14:1066–1072, 1997

Lustman PJ, Clouse RE: Treatment of depression in diabetes: impact of mood and medical outcome. *J Psychosomatic Research* 53(4):917–24, 2002

Madden PB: Diabetes and Depression. *Diabetes Spectrum* 23:11–40, 2010

Peterson K: Diabetes management in the primary care setting: summary. *Am J Med* 113:36–40, 2002

Polonski WH, Fisher L, Earles J, Dudley RJ, Lees J, Mullan JT, Jackson RA: Assessing phychological stress in diabetes. *Diabetes Care* 28:626-631, 2005

Ritholz MD, Atakov-Castillo A, Beste M, Beverly EA, Leighton A, Weinger K, Wolpert H: Psychosocial factors associated with use of continuous glucose monitoring. *Diabetic Medicine* 27:1060–1065, 2010

Rosenstock J, Ahmann AJ, Colon G, Scism-Bacon J, Jiang H, Martin S: Advancing insulin therapy in type 2 Diabetes, Previously Treated with Glargine Plus Oral Agents: Prandial Premixed (Lispro/ILPS) vs. basal/bolus (glargine/lispro) therapy. *Diabetes Care* 31:20–25, 2008

Rubin RR, Peyrot M: Psychological issues and treatments for people with diabetes. *J Clin Psychol* 57:457–478, 2001

Spilker B, Cramer JA (Eds.): *Patient Compliance in Medical Practice and Clinical Trials.* New York, NY, Raven, 1991

Stetson B, Schlundt D, Peyrot M, Ciechanowski P, Austin M, Young-Hyman D, McKoy J, Hall M, Dorsey R, Fitzner K, Quintana M, Narva A, Urbanski P, Homko C, Sherr D: Monitoring in diabetes self-management: issues and recommendations fo improvement. *Population Health Management* 14:189–197, 2011

Surwit RS, Schneider MS, Feinglos MN: Stress and diabetes mellitus. *Diabetes Care* 15:1413–1422, 1992

Turner RC, Cull CA, Frighi V, Hollman RR: For the UK Prospecitve Diabetes Study (UKPDS) Group. Glycemic Control with Diet, Sulfonylurea, Metformin, or Insulin in Patients with Type 2 Diabetes Mellitus: Progressive Requirement for Multiple Therapies (UKPDS 49). *JAMA* 81:2005-2012, 1999

UK Prospective Diabetes Study Group: Intensive blood glucose control with sulfonylurea or insulin compared with conventional treatment and risks of complications in patients with type 2 diabetes (UKPDS 33). *Lancet* 352:837–853, 1998

Wiesli P, Schmid C, Kerwer O, Nigg-Koch C, Klaghofer R, Seifert B, Spinas GA, Schwegler K: Acute psychological stress affects glucose concentrations in patients with type 1 diabetes following food intake but not in the fasting state. *Diabetes Care* 28:1910–1915, 2005

Wing RR: Behavioral weight control. In *Handbook of Obesity Treatment.* Wadden TA, Stunkard AJ, Eds. New York, NY, Guilford, 2002, pp. 301–316

Patient Selection and Goals of Therapy

Highlights
Patient Selection and
Goals of Therapy

Appropriate patient selection is crucial to the success and safety of any treatment regimen. A successful intensive diabetes management program must be a diabetes self-management program.

- Patient characteristics that influence success of intensive diabetes management are
  - willingness to be actively involved in care,
  - desire to improve glycemic control,
  - access to adequate diabetes education,
  - acceptable balance between treatment-associated risks and benefits,
  - ongoing communication with health care team, and
  - presence of adequate support networks.

- A successful treatment regimen is adaptable to meet lifestyle needs, balances the patient's risks and benefits, and is subject to ongoing evaluation and modification.

- No one set of glycemic goals can be applied to every person with diabetes. Glycemic targets must be modified according to the patient's age, disease duration, type of diabetes, prior hypoglycemia history, lifestyle, occupation, diabetes complications status, concurrent medical conditions, and support network. Health insurance status and adequacy of financial resources to cover health-related expenses may also influence the definition and subsequent achievement of glycemic goals.

- If intensive diabetes management is deemed unacceptable or inadvisable for a particular patient, efforts must still be made to encourage whatever degree of glycemic improvement is individually and safely possible.

Patient Selection and Goals of Therapy

Successful intensive diabetes management must incorporate diabetes self-management principles and strategies. The relative effectiveness of intensive management efforts is influenced by individual patient characteristics.

PATIENT SELECTION

Appropriate patient selection is crucial to the success and safety of any treatment regimen. However, the guidelines for patient selection cannot be rigidly defined. Instead, assessment of suitability for intensive diabetes management should be individualized and based on objective and subjective information provided by both the patient and the health care team (Table 5.1). All patients should be encouraged and supported to achieve the most intensified management they are capable of achieving.

Patients need to feel that they have options and that they are involved in the decisions that affect their health care. The health belief model (Table 5.2) offers some useful insights to consider when dealing with individuals who have diabetes.

Not all individuals with diabetes will be equally motivated to become more actively involved in their management. For some patients, injecting insulin once or twice a day or taking a couple of pills will be the maximum extent of their desired involvement. For these patients, it is crucial to determine whether their decision is an informed one, based on adequate access to objective information. After receipt of this information is confirmed, the continued decision to remain detached from self-care must be acknowledged and accepted by the health care team, while ensuring that the patient is neither neglected nor made to feel guilty for his or her decision. Motivation to improve self-care cannot be forced. Ultimately, the control of diabetes resides with the individual who has diabetes. However, health care providers are encouraged to acknowledge whatever positive changes are made and to continue to evaluate the patient for readiness to make more significant changes over time. Ongoing communication and education about diabetes management options and their benefits and risks may encourage patients to move toward more intensified management.

An individual's ability to make reasonable and informed decisions is influenced by knowledge of the pros and cons associated with each decision. Before committing to intensive diabetes management, the patient must be adequately informed of both the risks and benefits associated with intensive therapy. Decisions about the

Table 5.1 Patient Characteristics That Influence the Success of Intensive Diabetes Management Efforts

- Competent and involved in current self-care program
- Willing to become actively involved in daily management
- Desire to improve glycemic control
- Skilled in diabetes self-management techniques
- Accepting of benefits and risks associated with intensive management
- Willing to engage in ongoing open and honest communication with health care team
- Able to recognize physical and emotional abilities
- Has family or personal support for intensive diabetes management efforts
- Willing to use personal and health care support networks

appropriateness of individual patients for intensive diabetes management and discussions of the potential benefits and risks should be undertaken by a health care team that is not only knowledgeable about the pertinent literature related to intensive management but also experienced in its implementation. The health care provider must present a balanced review of perceived benefits and risks and avoid being judgmental or critical of the patient's decision to implement or not to implement intensive diabetes management.

If the commitment to improved glycemic control using intensive diabetes management has been made, the patient must have access to education regarding diabetes self-management techniques (see Chapter 3, Diabetes Self-Management Education).

In addition, the patient must be physically and emotionally capable of meeting the more rigorous demands of the intensive diabetes management regimen. Health care providers need to be sensitive to the fact that not all individuals will meet these demands in the same way. The patient's age and interpersonal support, as well as intellectual, emotional, financial, occupational, and domestic status, need to be taken into account when customizing an intensive treatment regimen and defining glycemic targets.

- Does the patient have the financial resources to pay for the increased costs associated with intensive treatment (e.g.,more frequent visits for medical care, education and counseling, testing, supplies, and equipment)?
- Is the patient self-sufficient or capable of assuming primary responsibility for daily care and treatment decisions?

Table 5.2 Health Belief Model

People are more likely to follow treatment recommendations if they believe that:
- They are vulnerable to the disease and/or its consequences.
- The disease could have a negative effect on their life.
- Following the treatment recommendations will reduce their risks.
- The benefits of the treatment outweigh its risks and/or costs.

- If the patient is not, is there a responsible individual who is willing to be educated and to actively participate in a more complex, time-consuming care regimen?
- If the patient lives alone, who will have daily or frequent contact with the patient in case of emergencies, such as severe hypoglycemia or illness requiring outside intervention?
- Does the patient's domestic and work or study environment permit and support the behaviors necessary to carry out intensive treatment?

Ongoing assessment of the patient's ability to achieve agreed-on treatment goals and integrate the regimen into daily life should guide decisions to alter the regimen. If any issues impair the patient's ability to carry out or monitor the effects of treatment, then regimen tasks, and/or treatment goals, including glycemic targets, should be modified.

A motivated patient and knowledgeable health care team collaborate to create a management plan with treatment methods and goals that are tailored to the individual. The regimen must be adaptable to meet the individual's lifestyle needs, must carefully balance the risks and benefits of therapy, and must be subjected to ongoing evaluation and modification. To ensure accurate and timely evaluation, the patient must be willing to commit to maintaining regular contact with the health care team. Through this frequent contact, effective changes can be made and problem-solving skills can be developed and reinforced.

For many patients, intensive management efforts enhance lifestyle flexibility and promote a sense of control over diabetes. However, glycemic control can be accomplished by many methods. Therefore, although modifications to an intensive treatment regimen may be necessary because of the patient's situation or for psychosocial reasons, glycemic control need not be sacrificed.

PATIENTS WITH TYPE 1 DIABETES

Intensive diabetes management should be considered for most individuals with type 1 diabetes. Implementation is strongly recommended for

- motivated individuals, with no early evidence of complications;
- women who are pregnant or contemplating pregnancy; and
- individuals with newly diagnosed diabetes.

Caution and care should be exercised when determining whether to pursue intensive treatment for specific subsets of the population with type 1 and type 2 diabetes (Table 5.3). All treatment decisions must weigh the benefits of the treatment against the associated risks, with the resulting balance dictating the individual treatment strategies and goals.

Many of the characteristics listed in Table 5.3 relate to patient difficulties with hypoglycemia, especially hypoglycemia unawareness or conditions predisposing to unawareness. Hypoglycemia unawareness has been considered an absolute contraindication to intensive diabetes management. However, in most patients unawareness can be reversed by meticulous avoidance of hypoglycemia for approximately 2–4 weeks. To determine the impact of hypoglycemia avoidance on hypoglycemia awareness, individuals with hypoglycemia unawareness or recurrent severe hypoglycemic episodes should be reevaluated after a rigorous attempt to

Table 5.3 Patient Characteristics That May Negatively Influence the Risk-to-Benefit Ratio of Intensive Management of Diabetes

- Hypoglycemia unawareness
- A history of recurrent severe hypoglycemic episodes
- Impaired counterregulatory response to hypoglycemia
- Use of medications that may interfere with hypoglycemia detection and/or treatment (e.g., ß-blockers)
- Other medical conditions that can be aggravated by hypoglycemia (e.g., cerebrovascular disease or angina)
- Severe emotional disorders or psychosocial stressors
- Alcohol or drug abuse problems
- Advanced end-stage diabetes complications
- CVD and longer duration type 2 diabetes
- Symptomatic coronary artery disease
- Cardiac arrhythmias
- Concurrent diseases and/or conditions that would functionally limit intensive management (e.g., debilitating arthritis or severe visual impairment)
- Relatively short life expectancy
- Age <6 years
- Inability or unwillingness to commit to the personal effort and involvement required for intensive diabetes management

prevent hypoglycemia for 2–4 weeks. Continuous glucose monitoring reduces the frequency of severe hypoglycemia unawareness by providing access to glucose trend information. If hypoglycemia unawareness can be managed or reversed, intensive therapy can be considered. The inability to manage or reverse unawareness indicates poor suitability for implementation of intensive therapy; however, efforts should be made to achieve whatever degree of glycemic improvement is safe and feasible.

Children, especially those younger than 6–7 years, require a team with special expertise and experience in the management of childhood diabetes. When such a team is available, intensive diabetes management is encouraged.

PATIENTS WITH TYPE 2 DIABETES

Intensive diabetes management should also be considered for most individuals with type 2 diabetes. Although the pharmacological treatment modalities may differ from those for individuals with type 1 diabetes, frequent blood glucose monitoring, nutrition management, physical activity, and ongoing communication with the health care team for assessment, education, care, and support are crucial components of the treatment regimen.

Current treatment strategies used in the care of individuals with type 2 diabetes require scrutiny. If patients are to accept the seriousness of their condition, their health care providers must review their personal management approach to type 2 diabetes and be cognizant of the message that patients receive. Statements such as "you only have a touch of sugar," "just follow your diet, and/or lose a bit of weight, and everything will be fine," or "you just have borderline diabetes" are counterproductive and will impede efforts to optimize glycemic control.

The myth that type 2 diabetes is a less serious, less debilitating disease than type 1 diabetes, because daily injections are not needed to sustain life, continues to influence and adversely affect treatment decisions. Several points must be made in this regard.

- Epidemiological data implicate hyperglycemia as a significant and modifiable risk factor for macrovascular disease.
- Nearly 40% of individuals with type 2 diabetes are treated with insulin.
- Despite the availability of numerous pharmacologic therapies, including those that specifically target postprandial glycemia, and the increasing use of evidence-based treatment algorithms and combination therapy, most patients are not achieving glycemic targets.

The patient characteristics listed in Table 5.1 also should be considered when assessing the appropriateness of implementing intensive diabetes management for patients with type 2 diabetes. Treatment decisions and goals must consider the presence and incorporate the management requirements of associated risk factors for macrovascular disease (e.g., hypertension, hypercholesterolemia, or weight gain). Special consideration should be given to individuals included in the categories listed in Table 5.3. These categories represent relative considerations, not absolute contraindications, for the implementation of intensive therapy. Again, if the patient is not an appropriate candidate for intensive management, efforts should still be made to improve glycemic control as much as is safely possible.

GOALS OF THERAPY

Before approaching the specific glycemic targets of intensive diabetes management, it is important to emphasize some basic goals of diabetes therapy (Table 5.4). It would be meaningless to set stringent blood glucose targets for the patient who is incapacitated by diabetes to the point of being unable to work or attend school because of recurrent diabetic ketoacidosis and/or severe hypoglycemia. For such

Table 5.4 Basic Goals of Therapy for All People with Diabetes

- Avoid life-threatening acute metabolic imbalance, including
  - severe hypoglycemia
  - diabetic ketoacidosis
  - dehydration
  - hyperosmolar hyperglycemic nonketotic coma
- Prevent hospitalization
- Minimize symptoms related to hyperglycemia
- Minimize symptomatic hypoglycemia that disrupts daily life and/or jeopardizes personal safety
- Maintain appropriate body weight (for all patients)
- Achieve normal linear growth and physical development in children and adolescents
- Accomplish normal school attendance, job performance, or social activities
- Experience a healthy psychosocial and personal life

patients, establishing a healthy, safe, and productive lifestyle should be primary. Specific normoglycemic targets should be attempted only after the more basic goals of reducing severe risk have been accomplished. Although some of these patients may respond favorably to intensive diabetes management, this is not universally the case. Patients with extreme swings in glucose levels may have poor psychological or psychiatric problems as a significant, if not primary, cause of their instability. Patients who have absent or blunted hormonal counterregulation are also poor candidates for stringent normoglycemic targets. Likewise, it would be inappropriate to set glycemic targets that could be accomplished only by interference with normal day-to-day activities (e.g., preventing normal attendance at school or on the job) either because of too many restrictions or because of excessive symptomatic hypoglycemia.

No single set of goals or target blood glucose levels can be applied to every person with diabetes. What might be recommended for an otherwise healthy young adult with type 1 diabetes early in the course of the illness may differ markedly from what is recommended for an older adult with coronary artery disease and reduced vision or for a toddler with working parents who spends most of the day in a day-care setting. Factors that play a role in determining the glycemic goals for any patient include age, ability to assume responsibility for decision making, duration of diabetes, type of diabetes, prior history of hypoglycemia, lifestyle or occupation, presence or absence of complications, other medical conditions or treatments, and availability of support from family or friends (Table 5.5).

GLYCEMIC GOALS

Data continue to support the pursuit of glycemic targets that are as close to normal as safely possible for each individual (Table 5.6). Target ranges for preprandial, postprandial, and bedtime glycemia serve as the reference goal for most patients with diabetes. However, these targets do not incorporate assessment of

---

Table 5.5 Factors to Consider When Establishing Individualized Treatment Goals

- Age
- Ability of patient to understand and implement a complex treatment regimen
- Disease duration
- Type of diabetes (type 1, type 2, or gestational)
- History of repeated or severe hypoglycemia
- Ability to recognize hypoglycemic symptoms
- Lifestyle and occupation (e.g., possible consequences of experiencing hypoglycemia on the job)
- Presence and severity of diabetes complications
- Presence of other medical conditions or treatments that might alter the response to therapy or prevent the patient from carrying out self-care behaviors
- Fiscal constraints
- Level of support available from family and friends

Table 5.6 Recommendations for Glycemic Control

Nonpregnant Adults

Glycated hemoglobin (A1c)	<7%*
Preprandial capillary plasma glucose	70–130 mg/dl (3.9–7.2 mmol/l)**
Peak postprandial capillary plasma glucose	<180 mg/dl (<10.0 mmol/l)

Postprandial glucose should be targeted if A1c goals are not met despite achievement of preprandial glucose goals.

More stringent glycemic goals (i.e., <6.0%) may further reduce complications at the cost of increased risk of hypoglycemia.

Conception/pregnancy

Preprandial capillary blood glucose *and either:*	≤95 mg/dl (5.3 mmol/l)	
1-h postprandial capillary blood glucose	≤140 mg/dl (7.8 mmol/l)	*or*
2-h postprandial capillary blood glucose	≤120 mg/dl (6.7 mmol/l)	

*Referenced to a nondiabetic range of 4.0–6.0% using a DCCT-based assay. Postprandial glucose measurements should be performed 1–2 hours after the beginning of the meal.
**Postprandial glucose measurements should be performed 1-2 hours after the beginning of the meal.

overnight blood glucose levels to mitigate the risk of nocturnal hypoglycemia. Most of the severe hypoglycemic episodes in the Diabetes Control and Complications Trial (DCCT) occurred overnight (43%) or during sleep (55%). A higher threshold for overnight blood glucose should be added to these goals. The frequently used value is a plasma glucose of 75 mg/dl (4.2 mmol/l). However, if the patient has a history of severe hypoglycemic symptoms or impaired cognitive function at blood glucose levels of approximately 60 mg/dl (3.3 mmol/l), then the nocturnal target level should be higher.

When practicing intensive management, some episodes of mild hypoglycemia are expected and considered acceptable, as long as they are well recognized and appropriately treated before severe hypoglycemia occurs and are not so frequent as to interfere with day-to-day life. Mild hypoglycemia becomes unacceptable when the safety of patients or those around them is placed at risk. For example, even mild hypoglycemia needs to be avoided during the operation of a motor vehicle or complex machinery or in those individuals with a reduced counterregulatory response to hypoglycemia (defective glucose counterregulation) or hypoglycemia unawareness. These conditions may occur as a consequence of recurrent episodes of mild hypoglycemia in some patients (hypoglycemia-associated autonomic failure) or as a result of autonomic neuropathy. Patients with complications that prevent recognition of hypoglycemia symptoms or recovery from hypoglycemia should avoid even mild hypoglycemia. Patients in whom it is determined that risky behavior or faulty decision making are contributing to frequent episodes of hypoglycemia should be referred for counseling or behavioral intervention. In most cases, monitoring strategies that significantly reduce risk can be put in place. If a patient persists in risk-taking, then the health care team needs to strongly consider altering glycemic targets and involving significant others in monitoring activities.

MODIFYING GLYCEMIC GOALS

Glycemic targets must be individualized. Specific situations requiring goals different from those shown in Table 5.6 are summarized in Table 5.7. Adults whose occupation requires continual mental alertness and quick reaction time for their safety or the safety of others need to be especially careful to avoid hypoglycemia. Adjusting glycemic targets to prevent adverse events should be considered. In addition, even in the absence of these specific situations, glycemic goals should be modified based on the level of understanding and motivation of the patient and his or her support network. Severe hypoglycemia, in particular, can be frightening to family, friends, and coworkers. Concerned individuals may insist on higher glycemic targets that ensure the patient's safety and may even actively sabotage efforts at intensive management when adverse consequences such as severe hypoglycemia recur. If a patient or family reports distress about recurrent hypoglycemic episodes, increasing the patient's glycemic targets should be considered and the treatment regimen reevaluated.

Pregnancy

A lower glycemic target range is recommended during pregnancy to improve outcomes. The American Diabetes Association recommends preprandial glucose levels ≤95 mg/dl (5.3 mmol/l) and either 1-hour postprandial levels of ≤140 mg/dl (7.8 mmol/l) or 2-hour postprandial levels of ≤120 mg/dl (6.7 mmol/l). Compared with intensive therapy in other settings, accomplishment of these targets requires more effort on the part of the patient and the health care team. Avoidance of recurrent or severe hypoglycemia must be considered in the pursuit of these stringent glycemic goals.

Children

The prior history of severe hypoglycemia and the potential danger for permanent neurologic sequelae associated with severe hypoglycemia need to be carefully considered when setting individualized glycemic targets for all children with type 1 diabetes. Children younger than 6–7 years are particularly

Table 5.7 Patients Who Require Alterations of Glycemic Goals

- Pregnant women and those planning pregnancy
- Patients with occupations in which the occurrence of hypoglycemia may endanger themselves and/or others
- Children <6 years of age with limited ability to recognize and effectively communicate symptoms of hypoglycemia
- Elderly patients, especially those living alone and those with cardiovascular disease
- Patients with a history of recurrent, severe hypoglycemia, or hypoglycemia unawareness

vulnerable to the long-term adverse effects of severe or repeated hypoglycemia. For young children with a developing central nervous system, significant hypoglycemia may be associated with a minor or, perhaps, even major loss of cognitive function that may be transient or permanent. We also know that hypoglycemia interferes with information processing, and repeated hypoglycemia may disrupt academic progress. Therefore, the avoidance of hypoglycemia is an especially important goal in this age group, and glycemic targets are higher than in older children and adults. For children younger than 6 years, the American Diabetes Association recommends preprandial glucose levels of 100–180 mg/dl (5.6–10 mmol/l) and bedtime/overnight values of 110–200 mg/dl (6.1–11.1 mmol/l). When a child can reliably report symptoms of hypoglycemia and take the steps necessary to obtain or carry out prompt treatment, premeal glycemic targets can be lowered to 80–170 mg/dl (4.4–9.4 mmol/l).

Premeal glucose values of 90–180 mg/dl (5.0–10.0 mmol/l) and values of 100–180 mg/dl (5.6–10.0 mmol/l) at bedtime/overnight are recommended for school-aged children (6–12 years of age). For adolescents and young adults (13–19 years of age), premeal glucose values of 90–130 mg/dl (5.0–7.2 mmol/l) and bedtime/overnight values of 90–150 mg/dl (5.0–8.3 mmol/l) are recommended. Postprandial blood glucose testing is indicated in situations where there is a discrepancy between the premeal blood glucose values and A1c, and to better assess overall glycemic control in those on basal/bolus insulin regimens. It is important to individualize the glycemic goals, with consideration of the risks versus benefits, and the capabilities and wishes of the family as well as the child.

Elderly Patients

Goals for therapy in elderly patients warrant special consideration. Many patients have other complicating therapies or medical conditions, such as cardiovascular disease. Some are visually impaired. Some live alone or have minimal support. Less-stringent A1C goals (such as 8%) may be appropriate for patients with a history of severe hypoglycemia, limited life expectancy, advanced microvascular or macrovascular complications, extensive comorbid conditions, and those with long-standing diabetes in whom the general goal is difficult to attain despite DSME, appropriate glucose monitoring, and effective doses of multiple glucose-lowering agents including insulin. The benefits of lowering blood glucose have not been studied in this population and may not be evident during the patient's lifetime. In addition to a less clear definition of benefits in the elderly population, the risks (especially those associated with hypoglycemia) may be greater. Assessing the individual's specific health characteristics and resources should inform the definition of appropriate glycemic targets to avoid increasing risk.

WEIGHING BENEFITS AND RISKS IN TYPE 2 DIABETES

The goals of therapy for patients with type 2 diabetes are similar to those for patients with type 1 diabetes. An individualized assessment of the risks and benefits of intensive management should guide therapeutic goals and interventions. Lowering pre- and postprandial blood glucose toward the normal range is desirable, especially in those with shorter duration of diabetes and/or absence of CVD. If this can be accomplished by regimens involving nutritional counseling, physical activity, oral or injected glucose-lowering agents, and/or simple insulin regimens (e.g., intermediate-acting insulin, premixed insulin once or twice a day, or a long-acting insulin once daily), then a more intensive insulin regimen may not be necessary. However, as the disease progresses, many patients will require the use of more aggressive or, perhaps, even intensive insulin regimens. The goals of therapy may require further modification because of hypoglycemia and/or additional weight gain. Many patients with type 2 diabetes are already obese, and weight gain may exacerbate their insulin resistance. For some, the risk of additional weight gain or hypoglycemia may outweigh the potential benefits of lowering blood glucose levels.

CONCLUSION

Improved glycemic control for all individuals with diabetes is the desired outcome of treatment interventions. The relationship of glycemic control and long-term complications must be considered in the context of the cost-to-benefit ratio associated with this treatment. However, if treatment strategies are to be effective in reducing long-term sequelae, then treatment goals and implementation techniques must be individualized. Not all patients will be able to cope with the demands of intensive diabetes management, but most patients will benefit from improvement in glycemic control. Failure to achieve glycemic targets should signal the need for reevaluation of self-care behaviors and regimen strategies. Encouragement to achieve any degree of improvement or increase in self-care efforts should be ongoing. Less than perfect glycemic control must not be viewed as a treatment failure or a character flaw.

No patient should arbitrarily be dismissed as ineligible or unsuitable for intensified diabetes management efforts. Instead, each patient should be critically evaluated for his or her ability and willingness to use intensive diabetes management, given the requisite knowledge, skills, and resources. In addition, if intensive diabetes management is reasonable for a given patient, but financial constraints prohibit implementation in the current health care setting, efforts should be made to refer the patient to community resources that may be available to assist the patient to achieve the most effective glycemic control possible.

Successful integration of an intensive diabetes regimen requires the melding of the patient's medical management requirements with the willingness and ability to perform the necessary treatment tasks. The health care provider is uniquely positioned to monitor, guide, and encourage the patient in the pursuit of glycemic control and long-term health.

BIBLIOGRAPHY

American Association of Diabetes Educators: The scope of practice, standards of practice and standards of professional performance for diabetes educators. http://www.diabeteseducator.org/export/sites/aade/_resources/pdf/research/ScopeStandards_Final2_1_11.pdf

American Association of Diabetes Educators (AADE): *The Art and Science of Diabetes Self-Management Education.* Chicago, IL, AADE, 2006

American Diabetes Association: Standards of medical care in diabetes. *Diabetes Care* 35(Suppl. 1) :S11–S63, 2012

American Diabetes Association: *Medical Management of Type 1 Diabetes.* 5th ed. Kaufman F, Ed. Alexandria, VA, American Diabetes Association, 2008

American Diabetes Association: *Medical Management of Type 2 Diabetes.* 6th ed. Burant C, Ed. Alexandria, VA, American Diabetes Association, 2008

Barker JM, Goehrig SH, Barriga K, Hoffman M, Slover R, Eisenbarth GS, Norris JM, Klingensmith GJ, Rewers M: Clinical characteristics of children diagnosed with type 1 diabetes through intensive screening and follow-up. *Diabetes Care* 27:1399–1404, 2004

Chase HP, Kim LM, Owen SL, MacKenzie TA, Klingensmith GJ, Murtfeldt R, Garg SK: Continuous subcutaneous glucose monitoring in children with type 1 diabetes. *Pediatrics* 107:222–226, 2001

Cryer PE: Hypoglycaemia: the limiting factor in the glycaemic management of type I and type II diabetes. *Diabetologia* 45:937–948, 2002

Cryer PE, David SN, Shamoon H: Hypoglycemia in diabetes. *Diabetes Care* 26:1902–1912, 2003

Diabetes Control and Complications Trial–Epidemiology of Diabetes Interventions and Complications (DCCT–EDIC) Research Group: Retinopathy and nephropathy in patients with type 1 diabetes four years after a trial of intensive therapy. *N Engl J Med* 342:381–389, 2000

Holman RR, Paul SK, Bethel MA, Matthews DR, Neil HA: 10-year follow-up of intensive glucose control in type 2 diabetes. *N Engl J Med* 359:1577–1589, 2008

Jacobson AM, Musen G, Ryan CM, Silvers N, Cleary P, Waberski B, Burwood A, Weinger K, Bayless M, Dahms W, Harth J, and the DCCT/EDIC Research Group: Long-term effect of diabetes and its treatment on cognitive function. *N Engl J Med* 356:1842–1852, 2007

Jacobson AM, Ryan CM, Cleary PA, Waberski BH, Weinger K, Musen G, Dahms W, and the DCCT/EDIC Research Group: Biomedical risk factors for decreased cognitive functioning in type 1 diabetes: an 18-year follow-up of the DCCT cohort. *Diabetologia* 54:245–255, 2011

Juvenile Diabetes Research Foundation Continuous Glucuose Monitoring Study Group: Factors predictive of use and of benefit from continuous glucose monitoring in type 1 diabetes. *Diabetes Care* 32:1947-1953, 2009

Kitzmiller JL, Block JM, Brown FM, Catalano PM, Conway DL, Coustan DR, Gunderson EP, Herman WH, Hoffman LD, Inturrisi M, Jovanovic LB, Kjos SI, Knopp RH, Montoro MN, Ogata ES, Paramsothy P, Reader DM, Rossen BM, Thomas AM, Kirkman MS: Managing pre-existing diabetes in pregnancy: summary of evidence and consensus recommendations for care. *Diabetes Care*:1060–1079, 2008

Maniatis AK, Toig SR, Klingensmith GJ, Fay-Itzkowitz E, Chase HP: Life with continuous subcutaneous insulin infusion (CSII) therapy: child and parental perspectives and predictors of metabolic control. *Pediatr Diabetes* 2:51–57, 2001

Martin CL, Albers J, Herman WH, Cleary P, Waberski B, Greene DA, Stevens MJ, Feldman EL: Neuropathy among the Diabetes Control and Complications Trial cohort 8 years after trial completion. *Diabetes Care* 29:340–344, 2006

Metzger BE, Buchanan TA, Coustan DR, de Leiva A, Dunger DB, Hadden DR, Hod M, Kitzmiller JL, Kjos SL, Oats JN, Pettitt DJ, Sacks DA, Zoupas C: Summary and recommendations of the Fifth International Workshop-Conference on Gestational Diabetes Mellitus. *Diabetes Care* 30(Suppl. 2):S251–S260, 2007

Nathan DM, Cleary PA, Backlund JY, Genuth SM, Lachin JM, Orchard TJ, Raskin P, Zinman B: Intensive diabetes treatment and cardiovascular disease in patients with type 1 diabetes. *N Engl J Med* 353:2643–2653, 2005

Nathan DM, Zinman B, Cleary PA, Backlund JYC, Genuth S, Miller R, Orchard TJ: Modern-day clinical course of type 1 diabetes mellitus after 30 years' duration: the Diabetes Control and Complications Trial / Epidemiology of Diabetes Interventions and Complications and Pittsburgh Epidemiology of Diabetes Complications experience (1983-2005). *Archives of Internal Medicine* 169:1307-1316, 2009

Nathan DM, Buse BJ, Davidson MB, Ferrannini E, Holman RR, Sherwin R, Zinman B: Management of hyperglycaemia in type 2 diabetes mellitus: a consensus algorithm for the initiation and adjustment of therapy – update regarding the thiazolidinediones. *Diabetologia* 51:8-11, 2008

Nathan DM, Buse JB, Davidson MB, Ferrannini E, Holman RR, Sherwin R, Zinman B: Medical management of hyperglycemia in type 2 diabetes: a consensus algorithm for the initiation and adjustment of therapy – a consensus statement of the American Diabetes Association and the European Association for the Study of Diabetes. *Diabetes Care* 32:193-203, 2009

Perranti DC, Lima A, Wu J, Weaver P, Warren SL, Sadler M, White NH, Hershey T: Effects of prior hypoglycemia and hyperglycemia on cognition in children with type 1 diabetes mellitus. *Pediatr Diabetes* 9:87-95, 2008

Peranti DC, Wu J, Koller JM, Lim A, Warren SL, Black KJ, Sadler M, White NH, Hershey T: Regional brain volume differences associated with hyperglycemia and severe hypoglycemia in youth with type 1 diabetes. *Diabetes Care* 30:2331–2337, 2007

Sacks DB, Bruns DE, Goldstein DE, Maclaren NK, McDonald JM, Parrott M: Guidelines and recommendations for laboratory analysis in the diagnosis and management of diabetes mellitus. *Clin Chem* 48:436–472, 2002

Silverstein J, Klingensmith G, Copeland KC, Plotnick L, Kaufman F, Laffel L, Deeb LC, Grey M, Anderson BJ, Holzmeister LA, Clark NG: Care of children and adolescents with type 1 diabetes mellitus: a statement of the American Diabetes Association. *Diabetes Care* 28:186–212, 2005

Skyler JS, Bergenstal R, Bonow RO, Buse J, Deedwania P, Gale EA, Howard BV, Kirkman MS, Kosiborod M, Reaven P, Sherwin RS, American Diabetes Association, American College of Cardiology Foundation, American Heart Association: Intensive glycemic control and the prevention of cardiovascular events: implications of the ACCORD, ADVANCE, and VA diabetes trials: a position statement of the American Diabetes Associations and a scientific statement of the American College of Cardiology Foundation and the American heart Association. *Diabetes Care* 32:187–192, 2009

Stratton IM, Adler AI, Neil HA, Matthews DR, Manley SE, Cull CA, Hadden D, Turner RC, Holman RR: Association of glycaemia with macrovascular and microvascular complications of type 2 diabetes (UKPDS 35): prospective observational study. *BMJ* 321:405–412, 2000

United Kingdom Prospective Diabetes Study Group: Effect of intensive blood glucose control with metformin on complications in overweight patients with type 1 diabetes (UKPDS 34). *Lancet* 352:854–865, 1998

United Kingdom Prospective Diabetes Study Group: Intensive blood glucose control with sulfonylureas or insulin compared with conventional treatment and risk of complications in patients with type 2 diabetes. *Lancet* 352:837–853, 1998

Whitmer RA, Karter AJ, Yaffe K, Quesenberry CP Jr, Selby JV: Hypoglycemic episodes and risk of dementia in older patients with type 2 diabetes mellitus. *JAMA* 301:1565–1572, 2009

Multiple-Component Insulin Regimens

Highlights
Multiple-Component
Insulin Regimens

- Multiple-component insulin regimens use four types of insulin.
  - The human insulin analogs lispro, aspart, and glulisine have the most rapid onset of action and time to peak effect and the shortest duration.
  - The intermediate-acting insulin Neutral Protamine Hagedorn (NPH) insulin (also called isophane) has a more delayed onset of action and peak effect and a longer duration of action.
  - The analog insulins glargine and detemir have the longest action profiles and are nearly peakless.
- Insulin absorption and availability are influenced by
  - Anatomical regions of injections, with the fastest absorption from the abdomen and the slowest from the thigh;
  - Timing of premeal injections;
  - Factors such as exercise, showering, bathing, and ambient temperature; and
  - Injection of insulin into areas of lipoatrophy, scarring, and lipohypertrophy.
- Multiple-component insulin regimens attempt to mimic physiological insulin release.
  - These regimens consist of various conformations of basal and prandial insulin components.
  - Frequent self-monitoring of blood glucose (SMBG) guides appropriate changes in insulin dosage and timing, food intake, and activity profile.
  - Prandial insulin is administered by syringe, pen, or insulin pump.
  - Basal insulin is administered with a rapid-acting analog by insulin pump or by injection of NPH, glargine, or detemir.
- Specific insulin regimens allow individual, flexible combinations of insulins and analogs that are suitable for various lifestyles.
  - Premeal regular or rapid-acting (lispro, aspart, glulisine) insulin and basal glargine or detemir insulin
  - Premeal regular or rapid-acting (lispro, aspart, or glulisine) or regular insulin and basal NPH
  - Continuous subcutaneous insulin infusion of rapid-acting or regular insulin
- Other insulin programs that offer less flexibility and generally less intensive management options are
  - Twice-daily mixtures of regular or rapid-acting insulin and NPH,
  - Prebreakfast rapid-acting insulin or regular insulin and NPH, predinner rapid-acting or regular insulin, and bedtime NPH,

- Prebreakfast rapid-acting or regular insulin, predinner rapid-acting or regular insulin, and glargine or detemir in the morning, evening, or both.
- Initial insulin dosages usually range from 0.2 to 1.0 units/kg body wt/day. Dosage requirements vary considerably during the remission or "honeymoon" phase (when there is residual beta-cell function), intercurrent illness, adolescence, or pregnancy.
- Insulin dosage is then divided into basal and prandial injections.
  - Forty to fifty percent provides basal insulin.
  - The remainder is divided among the meals, using insulin-to-carbohydrate ratios or preset dose guidelines.
  - All regimens must be individualized to the patient's desires, lifestyle, age, and defined target level of glycemic control.
- Insulin adjustments consist of an action plan for the alteration of therapy to achieve individually defined glycemic goals.
  - Changes are made in insulin dosage, timing of injections, or in the meal plan guided by SMBG results.
  - Pattern adjustments consist of modification in the current insulin dosage to minimize glycemic excursions throughout the day and to avoid hypoglycemia (<70 mg/dl).

Multiple-Component Insulin Regimens

This chapter discusses the design and use of insulin regimens for intensive diabetes management.

INSULIN PHARMACOLOGY

INSULIN TIMING AND ACTION

There are four general categories of time course of insulin action: rapid-acting (e.g., insulin lispro, aspart, and glulisine [genetically engineered insulin analogs]); short-acting (e.g., regular [soluble]); intermediate-acting (Neutral Protamine Hagedorn [NPH, isophane]); and long-acting (glargine and detemir [genetically engineered insulin analogs]). Table 6.1 summarizes the nominal action profiles—time to peak action and duration of action—of these insulin preparations.

A general pharmacokinetic principle is that a with longer time to peak, results in a broader peak and longer duration of action. Another principle is that with increasing insulin dose the breadth of the peak and the duration of action tend to be somewhat lengthened. The values included in Table 6.1 are for doses of 10–15 units, or 0.1–0.2 units/kg.

Rapid-Acting Insulin

Three genetically engineered insulin analogs designed to have a rapid onset and short duration of action when injected subcutaneously are currently available. Insulin lispro, [Lys(B28), Pro(B29)]-human insulin, contains an inversion of the amino acids at positions 28 and 29 of the B-chain. Insulin aspart, [Asp(B28)]-human insulin, contains a substitution of the proline at position 28 of the B-chain with aspartate. Insulin glulisine contains a lysine at B3 replacing asparagine, and a glutamic acid at B29 replaces lysine. These analogs have similar pharmacokinetic properties. They are sterile, aqueous, clear, colorless, and they have a neutral pH. In contrast to native human insulin, the modifications in the insulin molecule inhibit its ability to self-aggregate into hexamers and dimers in solution. This enables insulin to be more rapidly absorbed from the subcutaneou tissue after injection.

Table 6.1 Insulins by Comparative Action

	Onset	Peak Action	Effective Duration
Rapid acting			
Insulin lispro (analog)*	5–15 min	30–90 min	3–5 h
Insulin aspart (analog)*	5–15 min	30–90 min	3–5 h
Insulin glulisine (analog)	5–15 min	30–90 min	3–5 h
Short acting			
Regular (soluble)	30–60 min	2–3 h	5–8 h
Intermediate acting			
NPH (isophane)	2–4 h	4–10 h	10–16 h
Long acting			
Insulin glargine (analog)	2–4 h	Peakless	20–24 h
Insulin detemir (analog)	2–4 h	6–14 h	16–20 h
Combinations			
70% NPH, 30% regular	30–60 min	Dual	12–18 h
70% NPA, 30% aspart	5–15 min	Dual	12–18 h
75% NPL, 25% lispro	5–15 min	Dual	12–18 h
50% NPL, 50% lispro	5–15 min	Dual	12–18 h

*Per manufacturers' data; other data indicate equivalent pharmacodynamic effect (Plank J, Wutte A, Brunner G, Siebenhofer A, Semlitsch B, Sommer R, Hirschberger S, Pieber TR: Direct comparison of insulin aspart and insulin lispro in patients with type 1 diabetes. *Diabetes Care* 25:2053–2057, 2002).

Short-Acting Insulin

Regular (soluble or unmodified) insulin has the most rapid onset and shortest duration of action of any native insulin preparation, (that is, human insulin that is not modified to change its pharmacokinetic properties) with an onset at 30–60 minutes, a peak effect 2–3 hours after administration, and an effective duration of action of 3–6 hours. There is also inter-individual variation; in some patients, an effect is evident for up to 8 hours. Duration of action may be longer with large doses or when patients have insulin antibodies.

Intermediate-Acting Insulin (NPH Insulin)

NPH insulin uses protamine to retard and extend insulin action. The addition of protamine creates an insulin suspension, and after injection, insulin is more slowly absorbed from the subcutaneous tissue. NPH insulin has an onset of action 2–4 hours after injection, a peak effect 4–10 hours after administration, and an effective duration of action of 10–16 hours.

Long-Acting Insulins

Insulin glargine. Insulin glargine is a genetically modified insulin analog (21^A-Gly-30^Ba-L-Arg-30^Bb-L-Arg-human insulin). The amino acid asparagine at position A21 is replaced by glycine, and two arginines are added to the C-terminus of the B-chain. The effect of these changes is to shift the isoelectric point, producing a solution that is completely soluble at pH 4. When injected into the subcutaneous tissue, which has a physiological pH of 7.4, the acidic solution is neutralized. This leads to the formation of microprecipitates, or stabilized aggregates, from which small amounts of insulin glargine are slowly released. Glargine is absorbed from abdominal subcutaneous injection sites at a relatively constant rate, with no prominent peak in serum insulin concentration for 24 hours.

Insulin detemir. Insulin detemir is a long-acting basal insulin analog with a duration of action up to 24 hours. Insulin detemir differs from human insulin in that threonine has been omitted from position B30 and a C14 fatty acid chain has been attached to the amino acid at position B29. Insulin detemir is a clear, colorless, aqueous neutral sterile solution at pH 7.4. Its prolonged action is the result of slow systemic absorption of insulin detemir molecules from the injection site caused by strong self-association of the molecules and binding to albumin. Insulin detemir is more slowly distributed to peripheral target tissues because it is highly bound to albumin in the bloodstream.

Insulin Mixtures

There are commercially prepared, stable mixtures of regular and NPH insulins, insulin lispro protamine suspension (NPL) and insulin lispro, and insulin aspart protamine suspension (NPA) and insulin aspart. These mixtures contain either 70% NPH and 30% regular insulin or 70% NPA and 30% insulin aspart (called "70/30"), and 75% NPL and 25% lispro (called "75/25"). These premixed insulins may be helpful in elderly patients, blind patients, patients with cognitive impairments, or other patients who have difficulty mixing insulin in a syringe or using complex insulin regimens. However, because these mixtures limit flexible dosing, they are not useful for patients who desire flexible or intensive insulin regimens.

STABILITY OF INSULINS

Because insulin is stable for long periods when refrigerated, it is recommended that it be stored in a refrigerator. However, insulin is generally stable at room temperature for 28 days and does not need to be stored in the refrigerator after the bottle is opened, as long as it is used within this time. In contrast, insulin should not be exposed to extreme temperatures (e.g., in the car, near a window, or by a heating or air conditioning vent). It should not be exposed to direct sunlight or heat (including temperatures ≥30°C [≥86°F]) and should not be frozen.

Regular insulin and the synthetic insulin analogs (lispro, aspart, glulisine, detemir, and glargine) are all in solution. All other insulin preparations are in suspension. Vials containing NPH, NPL, and NPA insulin suspensions must be gently rolled at least 10 times (it has been recommended that pens containing NPH insulin be rolled and tipped 20 times), to ensure uniform suspension before insulin is withdrawn from the vial.

On mixing insulins, physiochemical changes may occur (either immediately or over time). As a result, the physiological response to the insulin mixture may differ from that of the insulins injected separately. Mixtures of two types of insulin vary in stability. Regular, lispro, aspart, glulisine, and NPH-type insulins are freely miscible in all proportions. These insulins may be mixed in the same syringe and their action profiles maintained. A decrease in the absorption rate (but not total bioavailability) is seen when insulin lispro, aspart, or glulisine is mixed with NPH insulin. However, most or all of the rapid action of regular insulin or the rapid-acting analogs is retained if mixing is done in a syringe immediately before injection. The acidic nature of insulin glargine precludes its mixture with other insulins. Also, insulin detemir should not be mixed with any other insulins because it can substantially reduce their absorption profile.

For reproducibility and to ensure equivalent dosing, it is important to follow a consistent routine from day to day. Patients should use the same technique for measuring insulin doses, mixing insulins, and administering insulin. If a patient is experiencing significant glycemic excursions after meals and needs a more rapid insulin effect, consider that there may be some loss of activity of regular insulin or insulin analog when mixed with NPH or its corresponding protamine analogue in suspension. This possibility can be tested by temporarily switching to separate injections. For patients who have their insulin premixed in a syringe by health personnel or a family member and saved for one or more days before use, ensure that an exception is not made on the day that the mixing is actually done. Namely, a visiting nurse premixing insulin for a week should mix the insulin for the day that he or she will next visit, so that all syringes have been stored for at least 24 hours before use.

INSULIN ABSORPTION

Many factors influence insulin absorption and alter insulin availability. Intraindividual variation in insulin absorption from day to day is ~25%, and between patients, is up to 50%. Although this variation is approximately the same (in percentage terms) for all insulin preparations, in absolute terms (minutes or hours), there is much less variation in absorption of short- and rapid-acting insulins and analogs and a greater variation in absorption of intermediate- or long-acting insulin analogs. Therefore, insulin regimens that use short-acting insulin or rapid-acting analogs are more reproducible in their effects on blood glucose.

Injection Site

There are regional differences in insulin absorption, especially for short-acting insulins (regular, lispro, aspart, and glulisine). Absorption is most rapid from the abdomen, followed by the arm, buttocks, and thigh. These differences are the likely result of variation in blood flow. The variation is sufficiently great that random rotation of injection sites should be avoided if possible. Patients should rotate injection sites within regions, rather than between regions, for any given injection, to decrease day-to-day variability. Because insulin absorption is most rapid in the abdomen (in the absence of exercise), it may be the preferred site for preprandial injections. Some patients use the abdomen for all preprandial injections, whereas others use the abdomen for the prebreakfast injection and other regions for prelunch or predinner injections.

Choice of injection site can influence the time course of any given insulin formulation and depends on the insulin regimen and the patient's lifestyle. For example, if an intermediate-acting insulin is used to provide basal insulin for a long period of the day (≥15 hours), it is desirable to inject into a site (e.g., the thigh) from which absorption is slow. In contrast, if the intermediate-acting insulin is used to provide basal insulin for a shorter period of the day (e.g., 8–10 hours), any injection site may be used. Moreover, if empirical evidence shows that the duration of action of any insulin preparation is longer or shorter than desired, a site may be chosen with faster or slower absorption.

Timing of Premeal Injections

Timing of preprandial insulin injections is crucial to matching insulin availability with glycemic excursions after meals. Insulin lispro, glulisine, and aspart have a rapid onset of action and should be given approximately 15 minutes before starting to eat a meal. However, if the meal is delayed, hypoglycemia may ensue. Subcutaneous regular insulin should be injected at least 20–30 minutes before eating a meal. The timing of injections should be altered depending on the level of premeal glycemia. When blood glucose levels are above a patient's target range, the interval between insulin administration and meal consumption should be increased to permit the insulin to lower blood glucose toward the target range. For example, when the premeal glucose is above target, rapid-acting insulin can be given 15–30 minutes and regular insulin 30–60 minutes before the meal. If premeal blood glucose levels are below a patient's target range, regular insulin should be injected immediately before meal consumption. Rapid-acting insulin analog administration should be delayed until after the patient has consumed carbohydrates and the blood glucose level has been restored to normal. In certain circumstances (if the ability of the patient to consume the meal is uncertain or if the quantity of carbohydrate in the meal can only be determined after its ingestion), it is acceptable to wait until immediately after completing the meal to administer rapid-acting insulin. The presence of gastroparesis diabeticorum may also significantly delay carbohydrate absorption and in these patients postmeal insulin administration may be advantageous.

Factors Influencing Insulin Absorption

Physical exercise increases blood flow to an exercising body part and accelerates absorption of insulin from that region. Sporadic exercise may induce variability in insulin absorption. The patient should try to avoid injections in a region that will be exercised while that injection is being absorbed. For example, if the patient intends to jog shortly after an injection, he or she should avoid giving that injection into the thigh. When exercise is contemplated, the patient might use the abdomen preferentially, because this region is the least likely to have significant increases in absorption (unless sit-ups are planned). Other factors influencing absorption of regular insulin are ambient temperature (e.g., a hot bath or sauna), smoking, and local massage of the injection site.

There is an increased risk of intramuscular rather than subcutaneous injection in thin patients with little subcutaneous tissue, which leads to more rapid absorption of any given insulin preparation. This can be averted by using short needles. Also, the interval between injection of preprandial regular insulin and meal consumption may need to be shortened. Some parents have reported that in thin, young children, insulin analogs are best administered immediately after a meal is eaten, both because of the very rapid onset and to ensure that the child has eaten before insulin administration.

MULTIPLE-COMPONENT INSULIN REGIMENS: GENERAL POINTS

There are two components of physiological insulin secretion: continuous basal insulin secretion and incremental prandial insulin secretion (Fig. 6.1). Basal insulin secretion restrains hepatic glucose production, keeping it in equilibrium

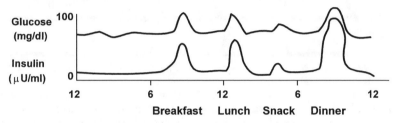

Figure 6.1 Schematic representation of 24-hour plasma glucose and insulin profiles in a hypothetical individual without diabetes.

with basal glucose use by brain and other tissues that are obligate glucose consumers. After meals, prandial insulin secretion stimulates glucose use and storage while inhibiting hepatic glucose output, thereby limiting the meal-related glucose excursion. Patients with type 1 diabetes lack both basal and prandial insulin secretion. Thus, insulin programs for type 1 diabetes require multiple components that mimic physiological insulin secretion by providing prandial insulin coinciding with each meal and basal insulin. Normal physiological insulin requirements include a background of basal insulin secretion between meals and overnight, combined with boluses of insulin coinciding with the rise in glucose that accompanies food ingestion with meals and large snacks. The most flexible regimens used for intensive diabetes management

- emphasize the need for preprandial insulin before each meal, separate from basal insulin;
- allow liberal food choices in terms of size, timing, and potential omission of meals while still balancing food intake with activity and insulin dosage; and
- include frequent monitoring of therapy to promote a more normal lifestyle.

Instrumental to the overall plan is self-monitoring of blood glucose (SMBG) multiple times daily. The patient takes action based on the SMBG results, which are used to help make appropriate changes in insulin dosage and timing, carbohydrate intake, and physical activity. The changes are made according to a predetermined plan provided by the health care team to the patient.

Prandial Insulin Therapy

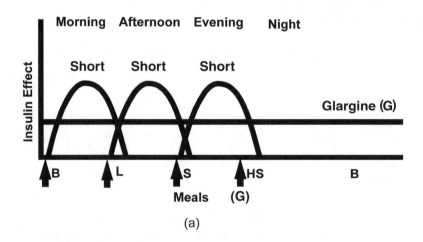

(a)

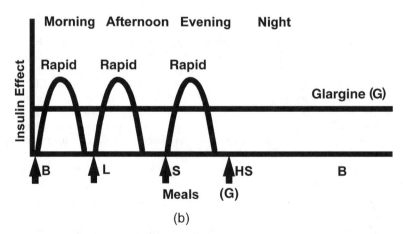

(b)

Figure 6.2 Schematic representation of idealized insulin effect provided by multiple-dose regimen providing basal long-acting insulin glargine (G) and preprandial injections of short- (a) or rapid- (b) acting insulin. Symbols: B, breakfast; L, lunch; S, dinner; HS, bedtime. Arrows indicate time of insulin injection. Although frequently given at HS, the basal insulin may be given at other times of the day and may be required twice a day.

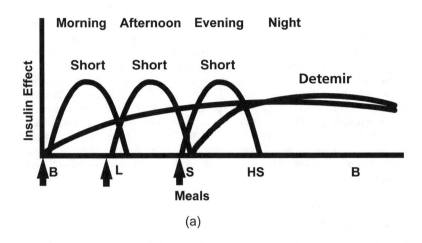

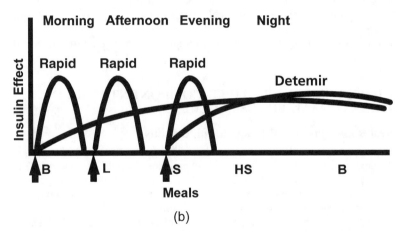

Figure 6.3 Schematic representation of idealized insulin effect provided by multiple-dose regimen providing basal long-acting detemir insulin and preprandial injections of short- (a) or rapid- (b) acting insulin. Symbols: B, breakfast; L, lunch; S, dinner; HS, bedtime. Arrows indicate time of insulin injection. Although frequently given at HS, the basal insulin may be given at other times of the day and may be required twice a day. Whatever the time of day that the basal insulin is given, it is best injected on a regular schedule approximately the same time each day.

Prandial incremental insulin secretion is best duplicated by giving preprandial injections of a rapid-acting insulin analog (lispro, aspart, or glulisine) before each meal by syringe, pen, or pump. Each preprandial insulin dose is adjusted individually to provide insulin appropriate to the current blood glucose level and the carbohydrate content of the meal. Thus, the size of the premeal insulin dose parallels the carbohydrate content of the meal. The timing of meals need not be fixed, and meals may be omitted along with the accompanying prandial insulin dose.

Regular insulin may also be used, but it is less convenient because of its longer time to onset and delayed peak relative to the analogs. Therefore, it is necessary to give prandial regular injections at least 20–30 minutes (or longer) before a given meal in an attempt to have prandial insulin parallel meal-related glycemic excursions.

Basal Insulin Therapy

Basal insulin is given as

- one or two daily injections of long-acting insulin (glargine or detemir), or
- intermediate-acting insulin (NPH) at bedtime and as a small morning dose, or
- the basal component of a continuous subcutaneous insulin infusion (CSII) program.

SPECIFIC FLEXIBLE MULTIPLE-COMPONENT INSULIN REGIMENS (BASAL–BOLUS REGIMENS)

Premeal Rapid- and Basal Long-Acting Insulins

This program uses three preprandial insulin injections of a rapid-acting insulin (lispro, aspart, or glulisine) and long-acting glargine (Fig. 6.2) or detemir (Fig. 6.3) insulin to provide basal insulin. If given twice a day, insulin detemir is a relatively peakless insulin. Glargine is also peakless in most patients when given once a day, and reaches a steady state 3–5 hours after administration.

Insulin glargine has a broad peak 15–18 hours after injection and a sustained action of 18–24 hours. It is sufficiently peakless to provide adequate daily basal insulin. If given with dinner, the waning effect after 18–20 hours may result in late afternoon hyperglycemia; therefore, bedtime administration may provide better coverage. For children who require snacks for adequate caloric intake, the addition of a small amount of NPH in the morning may obviate the need for administration of rapid-acting insulin at snack time. For young children, who require little basal insulin between 4:00 and 7:00 a.m., morning administration may be optimal.

Insulin detemir has a broad peak ~6–8 hours after injection and, when given twice a day, may have sustained action up to 24 hours. In most patients, twice daily detemir at steady state, has such a sufficiently blunted peak that it behaves as a peakless basal insulin. As a consequence of waning insulin effect after 20–24 hours, if detemir insulin is administered as a single morning dose, there may be an increase

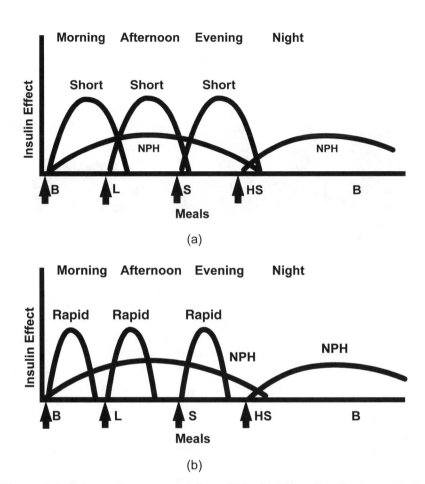

Figure 6.4 Schematic representation of idealized insulin effect provided by multiple-dose regimens providing basal intermediate-acting insulin at bedtime and before breakfast and preprandial injections of short- (a) or rapid- (b) acting insulin. Symbols: B, breakfast; L, lunch; S, dinner; HS, bedtime. Arrows indicate time of insulin injection.

in fasting glucose levels. Thus, it is best to divide detemir insulin into two doses. Alternatively, if used as a single dose, it should be given in the evening, either before dinner or at bedtime.

Premeal Rapid- and Basal Intermediate-Acting Insulins

This regimen uses three preprandial insulin injections (lispro, glulisine, or aspart) and intermediate-acting insulin (NPH) given at bedtime to provide over-

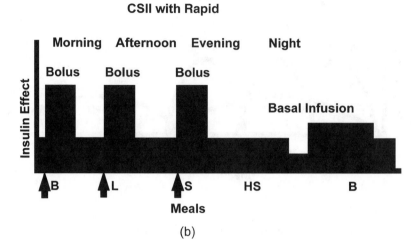

CSII with Rapid

Figure 6.5 Schematic representation of idealized insulin effect provided by CSII of rapid-acting insulin. Symbols: B, breakfast; L, lunch; S, dinner; HS, bedtime. Arrows indicate time of premeal insulin bolus.

night basal insulin with peak serum insulin levels before breakfast (a time of a relative increase in insulin requirements because of insulin resistance known as the "dawn phenomenon") (Fig. 6.4). Bedtime administration of intermediate-acting insulin also reduces the risk of nocturnal hypoglycemia. A small morning dose of intermediate-acting insulin (perhaps 20–30% of the bedtime dose) provides daytime basal insulin. Some patients may also need to include some intermediate-acting insulin before dinner and/or before lunch if there is a long interval between breakfast and dinner or between dinner and bedtime and the effect of the small dose of morning intermediate-acting insulin have waned.

This type of regimen has become increasingly popular in recent years for a variety of reasons. It offers flexibility in meal size and timing if the dose is adjusted. (If a pre-set dose is taken, the same amount of carbs need to be consumed.) It is also straightforward and easy to understand and implement, because each meal and each period of the day has a well-defined insulin component providing primary insulin action. If snacks containing >15–20 g of carbohydrate are required, as in the growing child or the pregnant patient, additional doses of rapid-acting insulin are required for these snacks.

CSII

The most accurate way to mimic normal insulin secretion clinically is to use an insulin pump in a program of CSII (Fig. 6.5). The pump continually delivers microliter amounts of a rapid-acting insulin analog (lispro, aspart, glulisine) , thus replicating basal insulin secretion. Moreover, to optimize glycemia, the basal rate may be programmed to vary at times of diurnal variation in insulin sensitivity that adversely effect glycemic control. Thus, the basal infusion rate may be decreased overnight to avert nocturnal hypoglycemia or increased to counteract the dawn phenomenon, which often results in hyperglycemia on waking. Temporary basal rates may be use and different patterns may be established corresponding to the needs of shift workers or persons having differing amounts of physical activity on given days.

The pump is activated before meals to provide increments of insulin as meal boluses. The meal insulin boluses are activated approximately 15 minutes before eating and whenever the meal is consumed. This allows total flexibility in meal timing. If a meal is skipped, the insulin bolus is omitted. If a meal is larger or smaller than usual or the carbohydrate content varies, a larger or smaller insulin bolus is selected. The ability to program the pump to vary basal rates over the course of the day and to suspend insulin delivery with increased physical activity, reduces the risk of exercise-related hypoglycemia. Patients should have syringes available for use in emergencies (for example, any time there is an interruption of insulin delivery due to a pump malfunction) and for times when they may find the pump inconvenient (e.g., during a day at the beach). For more on CSII, see Chapter 7.

OTHER INSULIN REGIMENS

Successful implementation of insulin pump therapy permits flexibility in eating and activity. However, such an approach requires a motivated, educated patient who is willing to carefully monitor blood glucose levels at least four times daily. Without motivation, education, or frequent blood glucose monitoring, an alternative approach is to maintain day-to-day consistency of activity and of timing and quantity of carbohydrate intake, thus permitting prescription of a relatively constant insulin dose.

INSULIN DOSE AND DISTRIBUTION

INITIAL INSULIN DOSES

In typical patients with type 1 diabetes who are within 20% of their ideal body weight, in the absence of an intercurrent infection or other cause of metabolic instability, the total daily insulin dose required for glycemic control is 0.3–1.0 units/kg body wt/day. The dose is lower during the remission or "honeymoon" period early in the course of the disease (e.g., 0.2–0.6 units/kg body wt/day). Moreover, during the remission or honeymoon period, because there is some continuing endogenous insulin secretion, it may be relatively easy to achieve near-normal glycemic control with virtually any insulin program.

During intercurrent illness, the insulin requirements may increase markedly (even doubling). Doses (in units per kilogram) progressively increase during pregnancy. Because the patient's weight also increases, the total dose may even triple. Insulin requirements typically increase throughout puberty and may reach 1.3–1.5 units/kg body wt/day, during the adolescent growth spurt.

INSULIN DOSE DISTRIBUTION

Approximately 40–50% of the total daily insulin dose is used to provide basal insulin. The remainder is divided among the meals, proportionate to the carbohydrate content of the meals. An initial dose of ~0.8–1.2 units of insulin for every 10 g of carbohydrate consumed is a reasonable starting place in adults. In children, the ratio of insulin to carbohydrate depends on age, body size, pubertal status, and activity level, with a range of ~0.3–1.0 units for every 10 g of carbohydrate consumed. The insulin-to-carbohydrate ratio should be individualized through the use of dietary intake records and blood glucose responses. Breakfast generally requires a slightly larger amount of insulin per gram of carbohydrate.

Alternatively, a constant carbohydrate diet can be prescribed with a fixed insulin dose based on the prescribed carbohydrate content (see Chapter 9). Some patients desire or require a dose of rapid-acting insulin to cover a bedtime snack.

INSULIN ADJUSTMENTS

Patients are provided with an action plan to alter their therapy to achieve individual, defined blood glucose targets before and after meals, at bedtime, and overnight. These actions are guided by SMBG determinations and daily records. Actions may include changing the timing of insulin injections in relation to meals, changing the amount or content of food to be consumed, and/or by altering insulin doses.

Two general types of adjustments are used: acute, usually preprandial, adjustments and pattern adjustments. The acute adjustments (also called corrective doses) provide an action plan that permits immediate action to be taken in response to current circumstances. Pattern adjustments provide an action plan that permits corrective action to be taken when a recurrent pattern is seen in blood glucose fluctuations. Attainment of therapeutic goals requires that both types of adjustments be used.

ACUTE ADJUSTMENTS

Acute adjustments may include changes in food intake and in timing of insulin administration, as well as changes in insulin dosage. In practice, most patients find adjustments in the insulin dose to be the most convenient adjustment to make. However, for especially low blood glucose values, additional carbohydrate is urgently needed, and for exceptionally high blood glucose values, a delay in the meal after the insulin dose may be needed. Many experts avoid the term "sliding scale," because the traditional sliding scale did not recognize ongoing (basal and prandial) insulin requirements and would prescribe no insulin when the blood glucose level was in the target range.

Acute adjustments are intended to correct momentary deviations of blood glucose outside the target range and so are frequently referred to as "correction doses." The correction may be used when there is variation in activity, intercurrent illness or other stress, or a need to correct variations in glycemia. The correction dose is in addition to the usual prandial and basal doses.

Corrections may actually be decrements (negative corrections, e.g., lowering of preprandial insulin in anticipation of postprandial exercise or in the face of prevailing blood glucose levels lower than the preprandial target). For patients on a constant carbohydrate diet, corrections (positive or negative) may be given for a larger or smaller carbohydrate meal.

Preprandial corrections provide an action plan for the patient guided by SMBG determinations and daily records. Calculations for corrective insulin dose are given in Chapter 7. One method of calculating the "correction factor" (the amount of additional insulin needed with a meal to restore the blood glucose to the target level) is to use the "rule of 1500": 1500 divied by the total daily dose of insulin is used to estimate the effect of rapid-acting insulin on the blood glucose level. For most adults, 1 unit of rapid-acting insulin will lower the glucose level 20–50 mg/dl. The correction dose is 1 unit per 20–50 mg/dl above the target glucose value. Thus, in a patient with a blood glucose level of 250 mg/dl and a correction factor of 1 unit per 50 mg/dl, the correction dose (also called the sensitivity factor) would be 3 units of rapid-acting insulin for a target glucose of 100 mg/dl. Obese patients with type 2 diabetes are typically insulin resistant and require a higher correction dose, as calculated by the above formula. The actions depend on the answers to several questions that the patient asks at the time of any premeal insulin injection.

- What is my blood glucose now?
- What do I plan to eat now (i.e., how much carbohydrate will I consume)?
- What do I plan to do after eating (i.e., usual activity, increased activity, or decreased activity)?
- What did I do in the past hour (i.e., usual activity, increased activity, or decreased activity)?
- What has happened under these circumstances previously?

The answers to these questions dictate the treatment response and become sensible routine decisions. The usual intervention is an adjustment in the insulin dose, but alterations in food intake (altering the amount or content of food), activity, and timing of injections in relation to meals may also be used.

PATTERN ADJUSTMENTS

Pattern analysis allows adjustment in the insulin dose when the blood glucose is consistently above or below the target range at a particular time of day. When a pattern is identified, action should be taken to correct the high or low blood glucose at that time of day (Table 6.2). The insulin dose (of the relevant insulin component most likely responsible) must be either increased or decreased to correct the pattern of glycemia outside the target range. Pattern analysis with insulin dose adjustments allows prospective changes to be made based on analysis of retrospective data. Pattern analysis can be especially effective when continuous

Table 6.2 Glucose Pattern Analysis Plan

This plan assumes that the prandial and bedtime blood glucose target is 70–130 mg/dl. Plans should be individualized for each patient.

Insulin assumptions

- Basal insulin (bedtime NPH, glargine, or detemir) is the major insulin acting overnight. Its effect is reflected in the results of blood glucose measurements during the middle of the night and on arising the next morning.
- Basal insulin (morning NPH, bedtime glargine, or bedtime or morning detemir) is the insulin acting in the later morning and later afternoon (i.e., >3 h after the premeal insulin dose).
- Prebreakfast rapid-acting insulin (lispro, aspart, or glulisine) has major action after breakfast. Its effect is primarily reflected in the results of blood glucose measurements 2–3 h after breakfast.
- Prelunch rapid-acting insulin (lispro, aspart, or glulisine) has major action after lunch. Its effect is primarily reflected in the results of blood glucose measurements 2–3 h after lunch.
- Predinner rapid-acting insulin (lispro, aspart, or glulisine) has major action between dinner and bedtime. Its effect is primarily reflected in the results of blood glucose tests 2–3 h after dinner.

Hyperglycemia not explained by unusual diet, exercise, and/or insulin

- If prebreakfast blood glucose is ≥130 mg/dl for 3–5 days in a row, increase basal insulin (bedtime NPH, glargine, detemir, or basal rate of insulin pump) by 1–2 units (0.05–0.10 units/h for CSII). (Before making such changes, verify that the blood glucose nadir, usually around 3:00–4:00 a.m., is not ≤70 mg/dl [<3.9 mmol/l].)
- If prelunch blood glucose is >130 mg/dl for 3–5 days in a row, increase prebreakfast short or rapid-acting insulin (regular, lispro, aspart, or glulisine) by 1–2 units.
- If predinner blood glucose is ≥130 mg/dl for 3–5 days in a row, increase prelunch short or rapid-acting insulin (regular, lispro, aspart, or glulisine) by 1–2 units.
- If bedtime blood glucose is ≥130 mg/dl (>7.2 mmol/l) for 3–5 days in a row, increase predinner short or rapid-acting insulin (regular, lispro, aspart, or glulisine) by 1–2 units.
- Increase only one insulin component at a time, starting with the one affecting the earliest blood glucose during the day.

Hypoglycemia not explained by unusual diet, exercise, and/or insulin

- If prebreakfast blood glucose is ≤70 mg/dl, or if there is evidence of hypoglycemic reactions occurring during the night, reduce basal insulin (bedtime NPH, glargine, detemir, or basal rate of insulin pump) by 1–2 units (0.05–0.10 units/h for CSII).
- If prelunch blood glucose is ≤70 mg/dl, or if there is a hypoglycemic reaction between breakfast and lunch, reduce prebreakfast short or rapid-acting insulin (regular, lispro, aspart, or glulisine) by 1–2 units.
- If predinner blood glucose is ≤70 mg/dl, or if there is a hypoglycemic reaction between lunch and dinner, reduce prelunch short or rapid-acting insulin (regular, lispro, aspart, or glulisine) by 1–2 units.
- If bedtime blood glucose is ≤70 mg/dl, or if there is a hypoglycemic reaction between dinner and bedtime, reduce predinner short or rapid-acting insulin (regular, lispro, aspart, or glulisine) by 1–2 units.
- Verify hypoglycemic symptoms with blood glucose measurements. Treat hypoglycemic reactions with 10–15 grams rapidly absorbed carbohydrate.

glucose monitoring (CGM) is used, either retrospectively to evaluate diurnal changes in glucose levels, or prospectively to aid the patient to make dose adjustments. These adjustments do not depend on the blood glucose at the moment when they are implemented. Instead, they anticipate insulin need for the future.

Glucose Pattern Analysis: Insulin Dose Adjustment

SMBG results should be analyzed every 3–7 days to determine whether there is a pattern to the results indicating a time of day when the glucose levels are consistently above or below the target range. The analysis can be broken down into the basal and bolus insulin components, looking first at the bolus component. If control is unsatisfactory, in case the bolus component exceeds 50-60% of the total daily dose, or in case the basal component exceeds 40-50% of the total daily dose, it may be appropriate to rebalance the apportionment of insulin between bolus and basal therapy.

Meal Insulin Pattern Analysis

To determine whether the meal insulin dose is appropriate, analyze blood glucose values 2–3 hours after meals. If the value after a given meal is ≤70 mg/dl (or the identified target) or ≥180 mg/dl (or the identified target), then that preprandial insulin dose should be adjusted until the postprandial glucose is in range. (See also Chapter 9, Nutrition Management.) If glucose levels are rising throughout the day and declining overnight without hypoglycemia, then the pattern of daytime rising may signal the need for upward adjustments of prandial insulin, especially if the prandial insulin constitues less than 50-60% of the total daily dose of insulin. A downward adjustment of basal insulin may be required.

Basal Insulin Pattern Analysis

After the meal insulin dose is established, analyze blood glucose values to determine whether the basal insulin is appropriate. The basal insulin should maintain the blood glucose levels in the target range from 2–3 hours after a meal until the next meal is consumed. The best patterns to analyze for basal insulin action are preprandial values (assuming the postprandial value is in the target range). If prepandial glucose levels, including prebreakfast levels, are high throughout the day without a marked upward trend in the course of the day, then the pattern may signal the need for upward adjustment of basal insulin, especially if the basal insulin constitutes less than 40-50% of the total daily dose of insulin.

Prebreakfast Blood Glucose Value

This value depends on overnight basal insulin, usually evening NPH, glargine, or detemir. If the fasting blood glucose value is below the fasting target, the bedtime insulin dose should be reduced in 1- to 2-unit decrements every 2–4 days until the glucose target is achieved. Results from continuous glucose monitoring indicate that glucose testing through the night, especially midnight to 4:00 a.m., is as important as the morning fasting glucose measurements to detect hypoglycemia. This is necessary to ensure safety of intensive diabetes management.

If the prebreakfast blood glucose value is above target, the basal insulin should be increased in 1- to 2-unit increments every 2–3 days until the target level is reached. Care should be exercised to verify that hypoglycemia is not occurring during the night when achieving a target fasting blood glucose level.

Prelunch Blood Glucose Value

This value depends on the prebreakfast insulin and either the evening or morning basal insulin dose. The rapid-acting insulin analog may not provide adequate basal insulin for the later morning. If the prelunch blood glucose value is above target (and the fasting and postbreakfast values are within target), additional morning basal insulin is needed. As the morning basal insulin is increased or added, the prebreakfast dose of rapid-acting insulin may need to be decreased to compensate for more morning basal insulin. A small dose of NPH insulin added to the prebreakfast rapid-acting insulin is frequently a more acceptable choice to the patient than adding glargine insulin, because it should not be mixed with a rapid-acting insulin analogs.

If the prelunch blood glucose level is below the target, the morning basal insulin will need to be reduced in 1- to 2-unit decrements until the blood glucose value is within target. If a decrease in the morning basal dose causes hyperglycemia later in the day, the addition, or alteration in the timing, of a morning snack may be considered for a slender individual or a young child, without reducing the morning insulin dose.

Predinner Blood Glucose Value

This value depends on the prelunch insulin dose and the basal insulin. If the predinner blood glucose value is above target, the fasting blood glucose and postlunch blood glucose levels are in target range, additional morning basal insulin is needed, or basal insulin will need to be added to the lunch dose. For some patients, especially growing teenagers, a dose of short- or rapid-acting insulin in the afternoon with a snack is the best solution for late-afternoon hyperglycemia.

Predinner hypoglycemia is seldom a problem with most regimens, but is resolved by decreasing the basal or the lunch insulin or adding a snack in the afternoon.

Bedtime Blood Glucose Value

This value most depends on the predinner insulin dose. However, if rapid-acting insulin is used and the basal insulin dose is delayed >3 hours after dinner, there is a basal component to this value. If the later evening blood glucose value is above target and the postprandial blood glucose is within the target range, some basal insulin is needed with the dinner injection. For growing teenagers who require additional calories in the evening, a small dose of intermediate-acting insulin added to the dinner dose may be helpful to avoid needing a separate rapid-acting insulin injection with the evening snack. For most weight-conscious individuals, the ability to omit an evening snack is a welcome advantage to rapid-acting insulin given at dinner.

INJECTION DEVICES

Making insulin injections easier and more comfortable assists patients to comply with a treatment plan. In particular, patients may be more willing to initiate intensive diabetes management if a multiple daily insulin injection regimen is made more convenient. Examples of injection devices include insulin pens and an injection port.

Insulin pens are especially useful in intensive insulin therapy. Insulin cartridges containing 300 units of regular, lispro, aspart, glulisine, NPH, 75/25, 50/50, or 70/30 insulin are placed in a pen-like device. Prefilled disposable pens are also available. Disposable needles (variable lengths available) are attached to the end of the insulin pen. The desired dose is administered by turning a dial selector, plunging the needle into the subcutaneous tissue, and pushing a button at the end of the insulin pen to inject the insulin. Insulin pens are convenient to carry in a pocket, purse, backpack, or briefcase and make insulin injections easy to administer away from the home. They eliminate the need to draw up insulin frequently throughout the day.

"Injection port" is the term used to describe small needles or Teflon catheters with an external port that can be inserted into subcutaneous tissue of the abdomen or other sites and remain in place for several days. Injections can be given through the catheter instead of through the skin, thus minimizing the number of needle punctures.

CONCLUSION

Intensive diabetes management involves flexible multiple-component insulin regimens tailored to the lifestyle of the patient. These regimens distinguish between basal insulin and preprandial insulin, using separate insulin components for different times of the day. Therapy is guided by frequent SMBG, at least four times daily. Patients follow action plans that guide them in daily self-management—altering insulin doses and timing, food intake, and/or activity—in an attempt to achieve the selected target level of glycemia. Patient education, collaboration, and motivation are critical to successful program implementation.

BIBLIOGRAPHY

American Diabetes Association: *Practical Insulin: A Handbook for Providers*, 3rd edition. Alexandria, VA, American Diabetes Association, 2011

Apidra [packet insert]. Bridgewater, NJ, Sanofi-Aventis U.S. LLC, 2008

Beaser RS, Blair E, Cooppan R: Using insulin to treat diabetes—general principles. In Beaser RS: *Joslin's Diabetes Deskbook, A Guide for Primary Care Providers.* 2nd ed. Philadelphia, PA, Lippincott Williams & Wilkins, 2007 pp. 249–279

Becker RHA: Insulin glulisine complementing basal insulins: a review of structure and activity. *Diabetes Technology & Therapeutics* 9(1):109–121, 2007

Bolli GB: Physiological insulin replacement in type 1 diabetes mellitus. *Exp Clin Endocrinol Diabetes* 109 (Suppl. 2):S317–S332, 2001

Cheng AYY, Zinman B: Principles of insulin therapy. In Kahn CR and Weir, GC: *Joshin's Diabetes Mellitus, 14th Edition*. Philadelphia, PA, Lippincott Williams & Wilkins, 2005, pp 659–670.

Colombel A, Murat A, Krempf M, Kuchly-Anton B, Charbonnel B: Improvement of blood glucose control in type 1 diabetic patients treated with lispro and multiple NPH injections. *Diabetic Med* 16:319–324, 1999

Danne T, Deiss D, Hopfenmuller W, Von Schutz W, Kordonouri O: Experience with insulin analogues in children. *Horm Res* 57 (Suppl. 1):46–53, 2002

Davidson J: Strategies for improving glycemic control: Effective use of glucose monitoring. Am J Med. 118 (Suppl 9A):27s-32s, 2005

Del Prato S: In search of normoglycaemia in diabetes: controlling postprandial glucose. *Int J Obes Relat Metab Disord* 26 (Suppl. 3):S9–S17, 2002

Diabetes Control and Complications Trial (DCCT) Research Group: Implementation of treatment protocols in the Diabetes Control and Complications Trial. *Diabetes Care* 18:361–375, 1995

Dornhorst A, Luddeke H-J, Sreenan S, Koenen C, Hansen JB, Tsur A, Landstedt-Hallin L: Safety and efficacy of insulin detemir in clinical practice: 14-week follow up data from type 1 and type 2 diabetes patients in the PREDICTIVE™ European cohort. *Int J Clin Pract* 61:523–528, 2007

Frid A, Hirsch L, Gaspar R, Hicks D, Kreugel G, et al: New injection recommendations for patients with diabetes. Diabetes &Metabolism 36:S3–S18, 2010

Gong WC: Determining effective insulin analog therapy based on the individualized needs of patients with type 2 diabetes mellitus. Pharmacotherapy 28:1299–1308, 2008

Grey M, Boland EA, Tamborlane WV: Use of lispro insulin and quality of life in adolescents on intensive therapy. *Diabetes Educ* 25:934–941, 1999

Hanefeld M, Temelkova-Kurktschiev T: Control of post-prandial hyperglycemia—an essential part of good diabetes treatment and prevention of cardiovascular complications. *Nutr Metab Cardiovasc Dis* 12:98–107, 2002

Heise T, Heinemann L: Rapid and long-acting analogues as an approach to improve insulin therapy: an evidence-based medicine assessment. *Curr Pharm Des* 7:1303–1325, 2001

Hirsch IB: Clinical Review: Realistic expectations and practical use of continuous glucose monitoring for the endocrinologist. J Clin Endocrinol Metab. 94:2232–2238, 2009

Hofman PE, Derrak JBG, Pinto TE, Tregurtha A, et al: Defining the ideal injection techniques when using 5-mm needles in children and adults. Diabetes Care 32:1940–1944, 2010

Hoogma RPLM, Schumicki D: Safety of insulin glulisine when given by continuous subcutaneous infusion using an external pump in patients with type 1 diabetes. *Horm Metab Res* 38:429–433, 2006

Kovatchev BP, Cox DJ, Gonder-Frederick L, Clarke WL: Methods for quantifying self-monitoring blood glucose profiles exemplified by an examination of blood glucose patterns in patients with type 1 and type 2 diabetes. *Diabetes Technol Ther* 4:295–303, 2002

Levemir [packet insert]. Princeton, NJ, NovoNordisk Inc., 2007

Mudaliar S, Edelman SV: Insulin therapy in type 2 diabetes. *Endocrinol Metab Clin North Am* 30:935–982, 2001

Peyrot M, Rubin RR, Kruger DF, Travis LB: Correlates of insulin injection omission. Diabetes Care 33:240-245, 2010

Ratner RE, Hirsch IB, Neifing JL, Garg SK, Mecca TE, Wilson CA, U.S. Study Group of Insulin Glargine in Type 1 Diabetes: Less hypoglycemia with insulin glargine in intensive insulin therapy for type 1 diabetes. *Diabetes Care* 23:639–643, 2000

Rosenstock J, Davies M, Home PD, Larsen J, Koenen C, Schernthaner G: A randomized, 52-week, treat-to-target trial comparing insulin detemir with insulin glargine when administered as add-on to glucose-lowering drugs in insulin-naïve people with type 2 diabetes. *Diabetologia*, 51:408–416, 2008

Rosenstock J, Park G, Zimmerman J, U.S. Insulin Glargine (HOE 901) Type 1 Diabetes Investigator Group: Basal insulin glargine (HOE 901) versus NPH insulin in patients with type 1 diabetes on multiple daily insulin regimens. *Diabetes Care* 23:1127–1142, 2000

Ruben RR, Peyrot M, Kruger DF, Travis LB: Barries to insulin injection therapy. The Diabetes Educator 35:1014-1022, 2009

Skyler JS: Insulin treatment. In Lebovitz HE: *Therapy for Diabetes Mellitus and Related Disorders*. 5th ed. Alexandria, VA, American Diabetes Association, 2009, pp. 207–223

Tsui E, Barnie A, Ross S, Parkes R, Zinman B: Intensive insulin therapy with insulin lispro: a randomized trial of continuous subcutaneous insulin infusion versus multiple daily insulin injection. *Diabetes Care* 24:1722–1727, 2001

Vajo Z, Duckworth WC: Genetically engineered insulin analogs: diabetes in the new millennium. *Pharmacol Rev* 52:1–9, 2000

Wolpert H: Understanding insulin: how it acts and how you respond. In *Smart Pumping for People with Diabetes*. Alexandria, VA, American Diabetes Association, 2002, pp. 111–124

Insulin Infusion Pump Therapy

Highlights
Insulin Infusion Pump Therapy

- Insulin therapy by an insulin infusion pump approximates physiological insulin delivery by continuously delivering a basal rate of short- or rapid-acting insulin and allowing bolus insulin administration before meals.

- For the motivated and capable patient with the necessary resources, insulin pump therapy is indicated for
  - suboptimal glycemic control,
  - wide blood glucose excursions,
  - dawn phenomenon with elevated fasting blood glucose levels,
  - nocturnal hypoglycemia,
  - frequent severe hypoglycemia,
  - pregnancy or planned pregnancy,
  - gastroparesis,
  - day-to-day variations in schedule that are not well managed by multiple insulin injections, or
  - patient preference for more flexibility.

- The basal rate should consist of 40–60% of the patient's total daily insulin dose. Several different basal rates can be set in a 24-hour period to accommodate diurnal variations in insulin sensitivity.

- Meal boluses are calculated based on carbohydrate content, using an individualized ratio of 1 unit of insulin per a specific number of grams of carbohydrate, usually 1 unit of insulin for every 10–20 g carbohydrate for adults and, for example, 1 unit of insulin for every 20–30 g carbohydrate for children or insulin-sensitive adults.

- The patient's insulin sensitivity or correction factor (ISF), which describes the effect of 1 unit of insulin on a patient's blood glucose level, is used to compute the correction dose of insulin that will bring premeal or between-meal hyperglycemia to glycemic target range. The ISF is individualized and is calculated using a formula. An alternative to calculating the ISF is to initiate an ISF of 50 mg/dl for adults and 75–100 mg/dl for children or insulin-sensitive adults.

- Patients can be taught to make additional adjustments in the basal rate and/or bolus size for illness, exercise, and menses.

- Risks of insulin pump therapy include
  - skin infections, which can be avoided or resolved with regular changes of the infusion set, by keeping the infusion site clean and dry, and by removing the infusion set at the first signs of discomfort or redness;

- unexplained hyperglycemia, usually resulting from a partial or complete interruption of insulin delivery that, if untreated, can lead to diabetic keto-acidosis; and
- hypoglycemia, which can be minimized by monitoring blood glucose levels at least four times per day, weekly at 2:00–4:00 a.m., and before operating a motor vehicle.

■ The insulin pump should be worn at all times. The patient should use an alternative insulin regimen if the pump is removed for >1–2 hours.

■ Successful insulin pump therapy requires thorough and ongoing education in technical components of the insulin pump and skills needed to adjust insulin for variations in daily activities.

■ Insulin pump theraphy in combination with a continous glucose sensor can improve blood glucose control without increasing hypoglycemia.

■ The future of diabetes treatment is promising due to advanced technologies that could lead to better information management systems, closed-loop insulin delivery systems, and further improvements in insulin pumps.

Insulin Infusion Pump Therapy

T he search for optimal insulin regimens led to the development of technology such as insulin infusion pump therapy, which helps patients achieve diabetes self-management goals. Insulin infusion pumps deliver insulin continuously in a manner that approximates physiological insulin delivery and provides flexibility in day-to-day diabetes management. Along with blood glucose self-monitoring, insulin pumps assist patients with diabetes to achieve near-normoglycemic control.

Continuous subcutaneous insulin infusion (CSII) consists of a small pump, about the size of a beeper or cell phone, that contains a reservoir of short-acting (regular) or rapid-acting (insulin lispro, insulin aspart, insulin glulisine) insulin. Most patients use rapid-acting insulin in their insulin pumps. After filling the reservoir with a 2- to 3-day supply of the prescribed insulin, the reservoir is connected to an approximately 18-to 43-inch length of plastic tubing. At the end of the tubing is a 25- to 29-gauge needle or a soft Teflon cannula that the patient inserts into the subcutaneous tissue at a 30- to 45-degree or a 90-degree angle, depending on the type of infusion set used.

The exception to this is the Omnipod® pump, which is tubing free but has a built-in infusion set in the pod for insertion into the subcutaneous tissue. With the Omnipod®, the patient injects insulin into the pod prior to placement of the skin and insertion of the infusion needle. The pod has a self-adhesive backing that attaches to the skin. The pod, like the infusion sets, must be changed every 2–3 days.

Insulin absorption is most consistent from the abdomen, and most patients find that placing the needle in the abdomen is simple and comfortable. However, patients can insert the infusion set in the hip, thigh, or upper arm. Infusion sets with a soft Teflon cannula are inserted using an introducer needle, which is removed after insertion, leaving the Teflon cannula in place. Teflon cannulas come in 6- to 17-mm lengths. Patients have a choice of cannula length and angle insertion, depending on their body type. Patients can also use a device provided by the manufacturer to assist in properly inserting these infusion sets. Most infusion sets have features that allow the patient to disconnect the cannula or needle from the infusion tubing either at the infusion site or inches away from the site, making it simple to disconnect the pump for brief periods, such as while bathing or changing clothes. Many infusion sets are also self-adhesive. After placing the filled reservoir into the pump, or applying the pod to the skin, insulin is continuously delivered into the subcutaneous tissue according to the rate(s) the patient has programmed into the pump.

The insulin pump delivers insulin in two ways. Basal insulin delivery is the continuous infusion of insulin and usually ranges from 0.4 to 2.0 units/h. Most patients achieve glycemic goals using one to three different basal rates over a 24-hour period. Depending on the model, insulin pumps can deliver basal rates from 0.025 to 35 units/h (in 0.025- to 5.0-unit increments) and can be programmed to give as many as 48 different basal rates in a 24-hour period.

Insulin is also delivered as a bolus, or larger amount of insulin, given in anticipation of a meal. Depending on the pump manufacturer, the pump can deliver a 0.025- to 80-unit bolus (most deliver a maximum of 30–35 units) in 0.025- to 2-unit steps. Patients can also administer a bolus to correct hyperglycemia that may result from illness, stress, or increased dietary intake. Insulin pumps can be programmed to deliver a bolus over a longer period of time, often referred to as an extended or square wave bolus. Patients can, for example, program their pump to deliver 4 units over a 3-hour period to accommodate snacking (such as at a party) or for a high-fat or low-carbohydrate meal. Patients can also program both a standard bolus and square wave or extended bolus at the same time, referred to as a dual wave or combination bolus.

Insulin infusion pumps have therapeutic and safety features that facilitate achieving treatment goals in different situations. Depending on the pump manufacturer, patients can use their pumps to

- Temporarily adjust the basal rate for periods of increased activity, illness, or stress without changing the usual basal rate program. The user can set the temporary basal rate in units or as a percentage of the usual basal rate.
- Suspend basal delivery if necessary. An "auto-off" is a safety feature that, if enabled, would suspend insulin delivery if no programming occurred within a specified period of time.
- Program several basal rate patterns (two to seven, depending on the pump model) so the patient can easily switch, for example, from a weekday to weekend pattern, premenstrual to postmenstrual pattern, high- to low-activity pattern, or day- to night-shift pattern.
- Review the amounts and times of previous boluses.
- Program boluses audibly or via a touch button or a short cut button that bypasses the normal bolus screen.
- Review total daily insulin delivery and alarm history; set the pump to beep or vibrate to signal alarms and alerts.
- Program different insulin to carbohydrate ratios, different insulin sensitivity factors, and different blood glucose targets by time of day.
- Prior to a meal, enter the number of grams of carbohydrate or exchanges into the pump or pump-linked personal digital assistant or manager (PDA or PDM), which is a programmable handheld device, so that the pump can calculate the amount of insulin needed based on the patient's personal insulin needs. Some pump systems have a food database from which the patient can select food items. Some pump-associated PDAs also have an integrated blood glucose meter.
- Use a pump-linked meter or continuous glucose monitoring system that transmits glucose values to the pump. The pump's bolus calculator can calculate the insulin bolus depending on the patient's insulin sensitivity, insulin-to-carbohydrate ratio (programmed into the patient's personal

settings), and time of last bolus . Most pumps calculate the amount of correction dose insulin depending on the time and amount of the previous insulin bolus to prevent "stacking" or overlapping doses of insulin. The duration of insulin action (usually 3 to 6 hours) is taken together with memory of the time and amount of the previous bolus to allow the pump to compute the "insulin on board" when the pump is asked to compute a new correction dose.

- Set a missed meal bolus alert to remind patients to bolus for a meal if they forget.

- Transmit stored glucose, insulin, and carbohydrate intake data to a secure website that can be accessed with permission by the health care provider.

- Pumps can come in a variety of colors or have "skins" in different patterns and colors that cover the pump and PDA or PDM.

- Set reminders on the pump to check blood glucose levels at specific times of day or if the blood glucose is above or below a specified level.

Insulin pumps have alarm systems for a low or dead battery, an empty reservoir or syringe, a low insulin level in the reservoir or syringe, an occlusion, or a pump delivery error; if a temporary basal rate is set; if pump delivery is suspended; and in the event of electronic malfunction. Pumps also have tamper-resistant blocks for added safety. Some insulin pumps are watertight or water-resistant so that patients can wear their pumps while showering or engaging in some water sports. Pump manufacturers specify the conditions under which pumps can be safely worn while exposed to water or moisture. Some insulin pumps can be programmed using a handheld device similar to a PDA, and others have a remote programmer. Many pumps have a backlight display that makes viewing the screen easier.

Many insulin pumps work in concert with a linked blood glucose meter or continuous glucose sensor. Insulin pumps and/or the PDA/PDM have bolus calculators that can calculate the patient's insulin bolus based on the blood glucose value, time of last insulin dose, and anticipated food intake if the patient enters this information into the pump or PDA/PDM. The calculations are based on the patient's own insulin-to-carbohydrate ratio, insulin sensitivity or correction factor (ISF), and duration of insulin, which have been previously programmed into the pump or PDA/PDM. The patient can choose to take or not to take the recommended bolus dose. Use of bolus calculators eliminate the need for the patient to manually make these complex and time-consuming calculations. Patients and their health care providers can use computer software to download all of the data stored by the pump and/or PDA/PDM. The software integrates history data stored in the pump with data stored in blood glucose meters, and provides data summaries and graphs for review and interpretation.

Insulin pump technology is constantly changing. Patients and health care providers should carefully evaluate the features of available pumps and determine which model best meets their needs. The pump manufacturer representative can provide information regarding the features of the pump and can facilitate payment from third-party payers. Pump manufacturers can also provide a diabetes educator who can teach the patient the technical information needed to implement pump therapy based on the health care provider's recommendations. Information regarding all of the insulin pumps is also available on the internet, where you can even see a demonstration of how the pump works through interaction with a "virtual" pump. In addition to the features listed earlier in the text, other factors to consider when selecting a pump are

- type, size, and placement of insulin reservoir (150- or 300-unit capacity);
- batteries (i.e., type, size, ready availability);
- weight, size, and shape of the pump;
- type of infusion sets compatible with the pump;
- warranty;
- availability of 24-hour technical assistance; and
- record of reliability.

The American Diabetes Association publishes a consumer guide every year in their consumer magazine, *Diabetes Forecast*, that provides current information on insulin pumps, blood glucose meters, and other diabetes management tools.

BENEFITS OF CSII

CSII therapy benefits from the pharmacological advantage of using only short- or rapid-acting insulin that is delivered as a continuous infusion, with incremental bolus administration at meals. This mode of insulin delivery most closely approximates physiological delivery. It also minimizes depots of insulin that are characteristic of conventional insulin delivery via a syringe, which can be mobilized by increased blood flow associated with exercise or warm baths. Short- or rapid-acting insulin is associated with the least variation in day-to-day absorption. The basal infusion allows patients to skip, delay, or alter meals without losing glycemic control. In addition, meal insulin boluses can be delivered during or after the meal is consumed, which may be beneficial for toddlers and children with unpredictable eating behavior and for patients with gastroparesis, or when consuming high-fat foods or meals that delay carbohydrate digestion.

Basal infusion rates can be programmed to coincide with the diurnal variation of insulin sensitivity. Patients often need lower basal rates during the night (between ~11:00 p.m. and 4:00 a.m.) and higher basal rates between 3:00 or 4:00 a.m. and 9:00 a.m. to offset the effect of the dawn phenomenon and prevent an increase in blood glucose levels in the morning. The basal rate can be adjusted temporarily during exercise, during the postexercise period when hypoglycemia is likely to occur, or during illness or before and/or during menses when insulin requirements tend to be higher. It is possible to program basal rates in half-hour segments throughout a 24-hour period.

Thus, insulin pump therapy optimizes the conditions for achieving good glycemic control while maintaining lifestyle flexibility. This therapeutic approach provides patients with the opportunity to fully participate in their self-care because they can make decisions about and adjustments to aspects of the regimen on a moment-to-moment basis as they encounter aspects of daily life.

Table 7.1 Patient Selection Criteria for Insulin Pump Use

- Medical/metabolic indications
  - Suboptimal glycemic control using multiple daily injections
  - Wide blood glucose excursions
  - Dawn phenomenon with elevated fasting blood glucose levels
  - Frequent severe hypoglycemia
  - Nocturnal hypoglycemia
  - Pregnancy or planned conception
  - Gastroparesis
  - Variable daily schedule/lifestyle not well managed with multiple daily injections
- Technical/physical ability
  - Perform blood glucose monitoring accurately and frequently (at least four times daily)
  - Perform the technical components of insulin pump use
  - Absence of serious disease or disability that would impair technical performance
- Intellectual ability (Patient must be able to...)
  - Learn the technical and cognitive components of pump use (e.g., meal planning, the meaning of blood glucose levels, and adjusting insulin)
  - Determine the relationship between aspects of the regimen (e.g., food and insulin, activity, and blood glucose levels)
  - Determine the relationship between behavior and outcome (actions and results)
  - Change behavior or aspects of the regimen based on the evaluation of outcomes
- Motivation (Patient must be willing to...)
  - Perform frequent blood glucose monitoring
  - Quantify food intake
  - Comply with recommendations for safe insulin pump use
  - Pay attention to aspects of daily life as they affect the insulin regimen and the needed adjustments
  - Anticipate insulin needs as circumstances change
  - Evaluate actions taken; engage in problem-solving behavior
  - Keep follow-up appointments
- Financial resources: Patient has a source of reimbursement for insulin pump, blood glucose monitoring supplies, and ongoing health care

Consider patients for insulin pump therapy

- to improve or stabilize glycemic control, especially if multiple daily insulin regimens have failed to solve self-management problems such as wide glycemic excursions, nocturnal or frequent hypoglycemia, and effects of the dawn phenomenon;
- to increase lifestyle flexibility and deal with day-to-day variations in work or exercise schedule; and/or
- to meet increased self-management needs (i.e., to allow greater participation in self-care).

Patients who have erratic schedules, work different shifts, or travel frequently can benefit from insulin pump therapy. Proper patient selection is critical to ensure the success of insulin pump therapy (Table 7.1).

INITIAL DOSAGE CALCULATIONS FOR
INSULIN PUMP THERAPY

Either rapid-acting (insulin lispro, insulin aspart, or insulin glulisine) or short-acting (regular) insulin can be used in insulin pumps; most patients prefer to use rapid-acting insulin. The rapid-acting insulin analogs have been used in insulin pumps without any loss of glycemic control and without an increased rate of hypoglycemia. The rapid-acting insulins have a quicker onset of action and a more pronounced peak of shorter duration than does regular insulin. Rapid-acting insulin should be administered 5–15 minutes before ingestion of the meal compared with 20–30 minutes with regular insulin. Peak effectiveness of rapid-acting insulin occurs between 50 and 120 minutes after dosing as compared with 2–4 hours for regular insulin. An advantage of using rapid-acting insulin in insulin pumps is that, when the bolus is administered an appropriate interval of time before a meal, postprandial hyperglycemia either does not occur or is attenuated. Furthermore, patients can more readily ascertain the effectiveness of the bolus because the peak activity is ~1–2 hours after dosing (although the effective duration can be as much as 5 hours). The rapid onset and 1–2 hour peak activity of the rapid-acting insulin can make correcting hyperglycemia simpler and quicker and lessens the likelihood that the action of boluses taken close together will overlap and lead to hypoglycemia. Most pumps calculate the amount of bolus insulin required depending on the time elapsed since the previous insulin bolus ("insulin on board") to prevent "stacking" or overlapping doses of insulin.

When switching from short- to rapid-acting insulin, frequent blood glucose monitoring is essential because the basal rate and boluses may need to change to accommodate the differences in the time course of insulin action. The patient may need a higher basal rate and smaller boluses with rapid-acting as compared with short-acting (regular) insulin.

BASAL INSULIN DOSAGE

The total 24-hour basal insulin is usually 40–50%, and is generally not more than 60%, of the total daily dose (TDD). Because insulin requirements may decrease with insulin pump therapy, if the patient has reasonably good glycemic control, reduce the prepump TDD by 10–25% before calculating a starting basal rate. A common mistake is to prescribe too much or too little basal insulin. If the basal insulin is <40% or >60% of the TDD, reevaluate the patient's insulin dosages.

For example, a patient with a glycated hemoglobin (A1c) level of 7.2% takes a total daily insulin dose of 55 units (reduce by 20%: 55 units × 0.20 = 11 units). Reduce the TDD to 44 units (55 − 11) and divide by 2 (total basal dose should be 50% of TDD: 44 units ÷ 2 = 22 units). Divide the total basal dose by 24 hours (22 units ÷ 24 hours = 0.92 units/h). The starting basal dose for this patient is 0.9 units/h.

An alternative method to calculate the total daily basal rate is to multiply the patient's weight in kilograms by 0.3–0.5. If the patient's weight is 176 lb (80 kg), the basal rate would be

$$(80 \text{ kg} \times 0.3 \text{ units/kg}) \div 24 \text{ hours} = 1.0 \text{ unit/h.}$$

Do several different calculations using these methods to determine the starting basal insulin dose. To avoid hypoglycemia it is advisable to start pump therapy using a conservative estimate of the patient's insulin requirement. Change the dose, as needed, based on results of frequent blood glucose monitoring and daily contact with the patient until desired blood glucose levels are achieved.

Most patients with type 1 diabetes require basal rates in the range of 0.4–2.0 units/h, with the average basal rate being 0.7–0.9 units/h. The average TDD for adults is 0.5–1.0 unit/kg body wt/day. Children will usually require lower doses of insulin, whereas patients with type 2 diabetes usually require more insulin.

Eliminate intermediate-acting insulin 12–24 hours and long-acting insulin 24 hours before initiating pump therapy. Instruct patients to take injections of short- or rapid-acting insulin, as needed, every 3–4 hours to keep blood glucose levels reasonably controlled until pump therapy is begun.

Patients using insulin pump therapy have the advantage of programming different basal rates for varying diurnal insulin needs. Patients often need lower basal rates between bedtime and 3:00–4:00 a.m. and higher basal rates between 3:00 and 9:00 a.m. to deal with the dawn phenomenon. Patients may need an intermediate basal rate during the rest of the day. An adjustment of the basal rate by 10–20% is usually recommended. Using the example above, if the patient's blood glucose profile revealed these varying diurnal insulin needs, the basal rate profile might be

- 11:00 p.m. to 3:00 a.m., 0.9 units/h;
- 3:00 a.m. to 7:00 a.m., 1.2 units/h; and
- 7:00 a.m. to 11:00 p.m., 1.0 units/h.

Evaluate the basal rate by the 3:00 a.m. and fasting blood glucose levels and with basal check tests (i.e., omission of a meal with glucose checks performed every 2 hours for a specific duration of time, usually 4–6 hours). If these values are higher or lower than desired, adjust the basal rate accordingly, usually by increments of 0.05–0.2 units/h. If the 3:00 a.m. and fasting blood glucose levels are widely discrepant, the patient may need different basal rates during sleep and in the early morning (before waking) hours. Adjust the daytime basal rate based on basal check tests. For example, if the patient develops hypoglycemia when meals are skipped or delayed, the daytime basal rate is too high. When using rapid-acting insulin, if the 2-hour postprandial blood glucose level is in the desired range but the premeal value is above the target range, the basal rate needs to be adjusted.

BOLUS INSULIN DOSAGE

Bolus doses are calculated based on the number of grams of carbohydrate consumed at each meal. Preferably, the patient starting a pump has demonstrated competence in counting carbohydrates for several weeks or months before the initiation of pump therapy. Ultimately, the patient should be able to match the meal boluses to the intake of carbohydrate at each meal and snack with an individualized ratio of 1 unit of insulin per specific amount of carbohydrate. This is termed the "insulin-to-carbohydrate ratio." A suggested starting ratio is 1 unit for

10–15 g carbohydrate for adults and 1 unit for 20–30 g carbohydrate for children or insulin-sensitive adults. For example, for a meal containing 60 g carbohydrate and an insulin-to-carbohydrate ratio of 1:15, the premeal bolus dose would be 4 units. Adjust basal rates so that snacks can be optional, depending on the patient's preferences.

During the first few days or weeks of pump therapy, it is useful to ask the patient to follow a prescribed meal plan based on the patient's usual dietary intake to establish the patient's insulin-to-carbohydrate ratio. It may be preferable to do this prior to initiating insulin pump therapy while the patient is using a multiple daily insulin injection regimen. Ask patients to keep detailed food records to help them master carbohydrate counting skills, demonstrate their ability and motivation to estimate carbohydrate intake and to determine their insulin-to-carbohydrate needs. Begin with a prescribed insulin dose for the meal plan, and make adjustments until blood glucose levels are in the desired range. When the patient demonstrates competence in counting carbohydrates, and the insulin-to-carbohydrate needs are established, the patient can calculate the amount of insulin needed for variations in dietary intake.

As with all insulin regimens and adjustments, frequent blood glucose monitoring must be performed to determine the effectiveness of insulin dosages relative to accurate carbohydrate counting and bolus calculations and to the patient's usual activity level. Blood glucose testing should be done, initially, before each meal, within 1–2 hours after the start of each meal, at bedtime, and at 2:00–4:00 a.m. until glycemic goals are achieved. Further adjustments will be required as the patient implements the insulin regimen under various situations. The patient should obtain a minimum of four daily blood glucose measurements (before meals and at bedtime) and a weekly blood glucose reading during the night around 3:00 a.m. once insulin needs are determined and target glucose levels are achieved.

Adjust premeal boluses based on the postprandial and next premeal blood glucose levels. For example, if the blood glucose levels 1–2 hours after breakfast and before lunch are higher than desired, increase the prebreakfast insulin-to-carbohydrate ratio bolus dose.

The patient's ISF is used to adjust boluses to correct for premeal and between-meal hyperglycemia. To estimate the patient's ISF, divide 1,500 (if using short-acting insulin) or 1,800 (rapid-acting insulin) by the TDD. For example, a patient whose TDD is 46 units has an ISF of 40 mg/dl based on the following equation:

$$1,800 \div 46 \text{ units} = 39 \text{ mg/dl (round up to 40 mg/dl)}$$

One unit of rapid-acting insulin is expected to decrease this patient's blood glucose by 40 mg/dl. Begin with a conservative estimate of the ISF.

A general rule-of-thumb starting point is that 1 unit of insulin decreases blood glucose 50 mg/dl (2.8 mmol/l) in adults and 75–100 mg/dl in children, but this decrease varies depending on the patient's insulin sensitivity and daily insulin requirements. For example, a patient whose TDD is 20 units may require only 0.5 units of insulin to reduce blood glucose 50 mg/dl (2.8 mmol/l), whereas a patient whose TDD is 80 units may require 2–3 units of insulin to decrease blood glucose by 50 mg/dl (2.8 mmol/l).

When determining the amount of supplemental insulin, the patient should be advised to consider the time of the last bolus. If using regular insulin and the last bolus was taken <4 hours ago, some percentage of activity from that bolus remains; therefore, reduce the supplemental insulin dose with that in mind (about 25% per hour). With rapid-acting insulin, peak pharmacodynamic activity is achieved in ~100 minutes, but duration is still a concern if the patient is calculating a between-meal correction bolus (about 33% per hour). If the pump is programmed to calculate the bolus needs based on the patient's ISF, it will compute the insulin dose needed based on the time of the most recent bolus ("insulin on board") to prevent "stacking" or overlapping insulin doses. The health care provider can program the pump for duration of insulin. For example, if the patient is using rapid-acting insulin and the pump is programmed for a three-hour insulin duration, the pump will automatically calculate a lower bolus dose if the previous dose was given less than 3 hours earlier.

Combining the insulin-to-carbohydrate ratio with the ISF, a patient with an insulin-to-carbohydrate ratio of 1 unit/10 g carbohydrate and an ISF of 1 unit/40 mg/dl would calculate a premeal bolus as follows (assuming the previous bolus was given beyond the programmed duration of insulin):

Blood glucose target is 110 mg/dl
ISF = 40
Blood glucose level = 179: 179 – 110 (target blood glucose) = 69; 69 ÷ 40 (correction dose = 1.725 units)
Carbohydrate intake = 60 g: 60 ÷ 10 (insulin-to-carbohydrate ratio is 1 unit/10 g) = 6 units of insulin
Calculated bolus is 6 + 1.7 = 7.7 units

The patient may need a different insulin-to-carbohydrate ratio and insulin sensitivity factor at different times of the day. For example, patients may be more insulin sensitive in the afternoon or after exercise. Different insulin-to-carbohydrate rations and insulin sensitivity factors can be programmed for various times of th day. If the patient is using regular (short-acting) insulin, the timing of the premeal bolus can be adjusted depending on the premeal blood glucose level. The effectiveness of regular insulin can be improved if the bolus is taken 45–60 minutes before the meal if the premeal blood glucose level is elevated.

INSULIN DOSAGE ADJUSTMENTS

DIET

Patients need to learn to adjust insulin boluses for variations in dietary intake so that blood glucose levels remain in the desired range. Usually 1 unit of insulin will cover 10–15 g carbohydrate. However, this can range from 0.5 to 2.0 units for every 10–15 g carbohydrate in patients with type 1 diabetes. Patients, with the help of their health care providers, will use food and glucose monitoring records to calculate the insulin-to-carbohydrate ratio, which may vary depending on the time of the meal (more insulin may be required at breakfast and less at lunch) or the type of food eaten. Precise estimates of the patient's insulin needs can be determined using detailed food, insulin, and blood glucose records. This is best done at the time the patient initiates intensive therapy when they are most interested in implementing their new therapy. Use detailed food records for a few days to a few weeks when initiating intensive therapy. Later in the course of managing insulin pump therapy, it can be useful to keep detailed food, insulin, and blood glucose records for a brief period, such as three days, to reevaluate the patient's insulin-to-carbohydrate ratio, and to review carbohydrate counting. This may be necessary if the patient's weight or circumstances change, or the patient's blood glucose levels exceed target levels. Patients can be taught to count carbohydrate exchanges instead of counting carbohydrates, and most pumps that have the capacity to calculate the patient's bolus can be programmed to count starch exchanges or carbohydrates.

A square wave or extended bolus can be used when eating small amounts of food over an extended period of time such as at a banquet or party, or when eating a high-protein, low-carbohydrate meal such as a steak dinner. Patients with gastroparesis may also benefit from delivering a bolus over several hours. Patients can also program a normal bolus and square wave or extended bolus at the same time (dual wave or combination bolus). This approach might be useful if a patient is eating a meal over several hours or is eating a meal high in fat, such as pizza, that can result in sustained, elevated blood glucose levels 4–7 hours after the meal. The patient might program a combination bolus consisting of 50% normal bolus and 50% extended bolus over 3–5 hours. If a correction dose is needed for a high premeal blood glucose level, give this portion of the bolus as a normal bolus. Blood glucose monitoring before and after the meal after several trials will determine the best dosing approach for a given type of food.

EXERCISE

Decrease the premeal bolus by 25–50% for moderate levels of planned postprandial activity. If the activity is strenuous, the patient may need additional carbohydrate. When exercising for sustained periods (>60 minutes), the patient may need to program a temporary basal rate reduction of 20–40%. A temporary reduction in the basal rate by ~25% after exercise for 6–12 hours may also be necessary to avoid postexercise hypoglycemia. Discourage suspending the basal rate. Yard work, shopping, and housework are activities that commonly result in hypoglycemia. Advise patients to reduce insulin for these kinds of activities. Patients who engage in unplanned exercise should consume additional carbohydrate without covering the snack with extra insulin. When using rapid-acting insulin, promptly reducing the basal rate for unplanned activity may eliminate the need for additional caloric intake (see Chapter 9, Nutrition Management).

Many pumps offer the ability to use a different set of 24-hour basal rates that are most effective for exercise. For example, for planned exercise at specific times, the patient may choose to "switch over" to his or her "exercise day" program, which the patient presets with lower basal rates at specific times.

ILLNESS

Patients using an insulin pump should follow the general sick day guidelines recommended to patients with diabetes. Insulin requirements increase during illness; therefore, if the patient has high blood glucose levels, increase the basal rate and/or premeal bolus by 20–50%. Adjust the basal rate so that blood glucose levels remain in a desired range overnight and during the day when patients cannot eat regularly because of the illness. Modify boluses to the patient's caloric intake. Frequently monitor the blood glucose and urine or blood ketone levels. Patients may need to take boluses of insulin using a syringe if they are unsuccessful controlling blood glucose levels using their insulin pump. If patients require oral or injected steroids, they should be advised that their blood glucose levels and insulin needs will sharply increase for a brief period of time. More frequent blood glucose monitoring will be required during these situations.

RISKS OF CSII

SKIN INFECTION

Skin infections can occur at the infusion site and range from a small area of mild inflammation and tenderness to a large area of induration, inflammation, and soreness with purulent drainage. Antibiotics usually completely resolve the infections. Large abscesses may have to be surgically incised and drained.

To avoid infection, keep the infusion site clean and dry at all times. Soap and water usually are adequate to cleanse the skin before needle insertion. Patients who experience recurrent infusion site infections may need to use antibacterial cleansers. Known carriers of *Staphylococcus aureus* require antibacterial cleansers and meticulous care of the infusion site and may benefit from antibiotic treatment. Patients should be instructed to remove moist tape and to clean and dry the area around the needle insertion site. This procedure is important during the summer or during increased physical activity.

Remove the infusion set every 24–72 hours and never reuse it. Subsequent infusion sites should be at least 1 inch apart, 2 inches from the umbilicus, and rotated to various locations on the abdomen. The cannula or needle should be comfortable at all times and should be removed immediately if irritation, redness, or inflammation occurs. Do not place the infusion set at the belt line or where constrictive clothing will cause additional irritation. Patients can apply a protective dressing to sensitive skin before taping the infusion set in place. An adhesive can also be applied to the skin before placing the tape to help the tape adhere better. If any redness persists or worsens, the health care provider should be notified promptly.

Patients sometimes report that insertion of the infusion set is difficult and/or that blood glucose levels are higher when the infusion set is placed in areas with scar tissue or where the underlying tissue feels hard or tough. Avoid these areas because insulin absorption may be poor or unpredictable. Use alternative sites such as the hip or thigh until the tissue has healed.

There are several types of infusion sets with various cannula and needle types, including straight or angled needles, needles attached to an adhesive disk, and Teflon cannulas with needle introducers. Small devices are available that make it

Table 7.2 Unexplained Hyperglycemia: Factors to Consider

- Insulin pump
  - Basal rate programmed incorrectly
  - Battery depleted
  - Pump malfunction
  - Cartridge or syringe (reservoir) does not advance properly/pod is not functioning
  - Program and/or pump alarms
  - Program functions cannot be set
- Cartridge or syringe (reservoir)
  - Improper placement in the pump
  - Empty cartridge or syringe (insulin depleted)
  - Leakage of insulin
  - Cartridge or syringe not positioned to advance and infuse
  - Did not prime reservoir or infusion set correctly
- Infusion set and needle or cannula
  - Insulin leakage
  - Dislodged needle, cannula, or pod
  - Bent or kinked cannula or incorrect cannula or pod insertion
  - Insulin not administered to account for dead space after introducer needle is removed when infusion cannula is inserted
  - Air in infusion set tubing
  - Blood in infusion set tubing
  - Occlusion at the site
  - Infusion set in place >48–72 h
  - Tear in the tubing
  - Occlusion of the insulin in the infusion set
  - Loose cartridge or syringe and infusion set connection
- Infusion site
  - Redness, irritation, inflammation, induration
  - Discomfort
  - Placement in an area of hypertrophy or scar tissue
  - Placement in an area of friction or near the belt line
- Insulin
  - Not buffered
  - Has clumped particles or crystallized appearance
  - Is beyond expiration date
  - Was exposed to extreme temperatures
  - Vial has been used for >1 month or is nearly empty
- Patient
  - Prior bolus omitted
  - Prior bolus inadequate for carbohydrate consumed

easier for the patient to correctly insert the needle introducers. Infusion sets are available with a disconnect feature that allows the patient to easily disconnect from the pump without removing the infusion set. Most cannula or infusion site problems, such as difficulty with needle insertion and skin breakdown, can be resolved by finding the type of cannula and tape/adhesive that best suits the individual patient.

Most infusion sets have self-adhesive tape; use of an additional adhesive dressing or surgical tape can help secure the needle or cannula and tubing in place. If patients are allergic to the self-adhesive infusion sets, find a tape or surgical dressing that does not cause a skin reaction, or have the patient apply a protective solution or dressing (I.V. Prep Antiseptic Wipe, Tegaderm™, Skin-Tac™, Bard Protective Barrier Film®, Mastisol®, or Skin Bond™) before inserting the infusion set. Consult the pump manufacturer for specific product information. Most pumps are compatible with many of the manufacturer's infusion sets.

UNEXPLAINED HYPERGLYCEMIA AND KETOACIDOSIS

Because the insulin pump only uses rapid- or short-acting insulin, even a partial interruption of insulin delivery can rapidly result in hyperglycemia. Complete interruption of insulin delivery can result in ketosis or ketoacidosis within a few hours.

Patients new to insulin pump therapy must be taught to consider the possibility of interrupted insulin delivery any time high blood glucose levels persist for no apparent reason. In the absence of illness, if there has been no increase in dietary intake, no change in the insulin dose or timing, or no alteration in stress or activity levels, a disruption in insulin delivery should be suspected if hyperglycemia persists. The first indication of unexplained hyperglycemia often occurs with a routine blood glucose test, when the patient is surprised by an unusually high blood glucose value. If the blood glucose level has not decreased 2–4 hours later after administering a correction bolus, hyperglycemia caused by an interruption of insulin delivery is the likely cause. If urine ketones are also present or blood ketone (beta-hydroxybutyrate) levels are increased, a disruption of insulin delivery must be considered. Sometimes, the cause of unexplained hyperglycemia is insulin that has lost potency. This should be suspected if no improvement in blood glucose levels are seen when the patient changes the reservoir and infusion set. If the patient administers an insulin bolus via a conventional syringe and the blood glucose level improves, there is a problem with the insulin pump and/or the reservoir/pod, and not with the insulin.

There are many potential causes of unexplained hyperglycemia or ketoacidosis related to partial or complete failure of some component of the insulin infusion pump, syringe, and/or infusion set/pod (Table 7.2). When a patient encounters a high blood glucose level (>250 mg/dl [>13.8 mmol/l]) that cannot be explained by an alteration in a component of the treatment plan, the patient should do a systematic investigation of the pump, cartridge or syringe, infusion set/pod, infusion site, and insulin to identify the cause. If the patient detects a problem with the site, the infusion set tubing, or the connection between the syringe and the infusion set, immediately change the cannula/pod and site. If a problem with the pump is identified, reprogram the pump or contact the pump manufacturer to troubleshoot the problem or have the pump replaced if it is within the warranty period. Patients need to use insulin injections until the pump is replaced. If the cartridge or syringe or insulin is faulty, change the insulin, syringe, infusion set, and site. Make sure the patient primes the infusion set properly before inserting the infusion set (filling the infusion set and, if using a nondisconnect needle or cannula, filling the needle or cannula with insulin before insertion into the subcutaneous tissue). If using a disconnect infusion set, the patient must be sure to fill the subcutaneous cannula after connecting the tubing or after removing the needle introducer when using an infusion set that uses a Teflon cannula. Each infusion set

Table 7.3 Education for Insulin Pump Therapy

Phase 1: Choosing insulin pump therapy (1–2 outpatient visits)

- Components of insulin pump therapy
- Advantages and disadvantages of insulin pump therapy
- Financial requirements
- Goals of therapy
- Carbohydrate counting (minimum two sessions)
- Suitability for insulin pump use (e.g., several-month trial of frequent blood glucose monitoring, trial of multiple daily insulin injections, carbohydrate counting, and use of insulin sensitivity/correction factor)

Phase 2: Initiating insulin pump therapy

- Several sessions with health care team over several months, a 2- to 4-h technical training session with pump trainer, and a visit with health care provider
- Technical components of the insulin pump (Table 7.4)
- Blood glucose–monitoring technique and accuracy confirmed
- Carbohydrate counting review and fine-tuning to establish insulin-to-carbohydrate ratio
- Symptoms, prevention, and treatment of hypoglycemia
- Optional trial of wearing the insulin pump using normal saline
- Determination of initial starting basal rate

Phase 3: Post-initiation of insulin pump therapy

- Daily phone contact for 7–10 days and biweekly follow-up visits for first 2–4 weeks; maintain close contact for 2–6 months; have patient keep food, blood glucose, and insulin records
- Focus on mastering blood glucose monitoring, calculating meal boluses based on carbohydrate counting, calculating correction bolus doses based on glucose monitoring, and insulin pump operation
- Fine-tune insulin dosages to achieve blood glucose goals
- Identify relationships between blood glucose readings and food intake, activity, and insulin
- Adjust aspects of the regimen to meet lifestyle needs based on patient input
- Assist patient to integrate the treatment plan into daily life

Ongoing follow-up

- Visits every 1–3 months of 30–60 min using all team members as needed
- Interpreting blood glucose readings
- Adjusting insulin for variations in dietary intake and activity
- Using the pump and advanced pump options to deal with varying situations
- Dealing with pump-related problems
- Adapting treatment recommendations to changes in lifestyle
- Anticipating situations that could cause alterations in glycemic control
- Identifying obstacles to implementing treatment recommendations and developing strategies to overcome obstacles
- Setting and evaluating treatment and blood glucose goals

has instructions detailing the amount of insulin needed to fill the cannula after the introducer needle is removed.

If no obvious cause is found, assume that there is an infusion problem, most likely caused by a partial or complete occlusion of insulin in the infusion set or at the infusion site, and replace the cartridge or syringe and infusion set or pod and change the site. Sometimes insulin loses potency and simply using a new vial of insulin will correct the problem.

If the pump is inoperable or malfunctioning, patients should use a multiple-injection regimen until the pump can be replaced (see Chapter 6). All patients should know how to use an alternative insulin regimen with conventional insulin syringes in case a problem with the pump or some component of the infusion system occurs. Instruct patients to always carry extra insulin, pump supplies (batteries, infusion sets, and pump cartridges, syringes, or pods), and conventional syringes or an insulin pen delivery device. If a pump malfunction is suspected, the patient should contact the health care provider. The patient can also obtain technical assistance from the pump manufacturer.

When the patient detects unexplained hyperglycemia and corrects the problem, then the hyperglycemia and ketonuria must be treated. The patient should monitor blood glucose and urine or blood ketone levels every 1–3 hours. Advise the patient to take insulin boluses in amounts determined by the patient's insulin sensitivity and daily insulin requirements until urine ketones have cleared (or blood ketone levels are <0.6 mmol/l) and blood glucose levels have returned to the desired range. The patient should take insulin via conventional injections to correct the hyperglycemia and ketosis, especially if pump malfunction is suspected. The patient who develops nausea and vomiting and is unable to maintain fluid intake should go to an emergency room for treatment.

Reduce the incidence of unexplained hyperglycemia by following a few guidelines. Change infusion sets/pods at least every 24–72 hours. If blood appears in the tubing, replace the infusion set/pod immediately because the blood may clot and block insulin delivery. Ideally, insert the infusion set/pod before the administration of a bolus to lessen the possibility that tissue will clog the needle or cannula. Insert the infusion set/pod at a time of day when the blood glucose level can be checked 2 hours later to make sure that insulin is being properly delivered (do not insert the infusion set/pod at bedtime). Do not insert the infusion set/pod into scar tissue or into tissue that is hard or tough. Do not remove the infusion set/pod soon after delivering a bolus because insulin can pool at the site and the patient might not get the full bolus. If there are air bubbles in the tubing, disconnect the tubing from the needle or cannula and use the prime, fill or bolus feature to push the air out. Ketosis and/or ketoacidosis can be completely avoided if patients monitor blood glucose levels frequently and correct unexplained hyperglycemia as soon as it occurs.

HYPOGLYCEMIA

A lower incidence of hypoglycemia has been observed with insulin pump therapy as compared to multiple daily injections. Strategies for avoiding hypoglycemia and methods of teaching hypoglycemia awareness are essentially the same for any intensive diabetes management approach, regardless of the mode of insulin delivery. Patients should have a source of rapidly absorbed carbohydrate such as juice, regular soda, or glucose tablets with them at all times, including at work, in the car, at the gym, and at the bedside. Encourage patients to check their blood glucose levels before operating machinery or a motor vehicle. All patients using a pump should have glucagon and a close family member or friend instructed on its use. To avoid accidentally infusing insulin, advise patients to disconnect the infusion set tubing before removing a used cartridge or reservoir (syringe) or replacing an infusion set. The patient should not use the prime, load, or fill tubing feature while an infusion set is connected to the body. All caregivers, including family members, school personnel, and daycare providers, should know how to troubleshoot pump problems, including how to suspend pump operation in the event of severe hypoglycemia.

Avoiding severe hypoglycemia begins with selecting patients who are good candidates for intensive therapy (Table 7.3). Patients must be prepared to check blood glucose levels at least four times a day to monitor pump operation and to make and evaluate decisions regarding insulin doses. Patients often take insulin without checking their blood glucose levels, a practice that increases the risk of hypoglycemia. This should be discouraged. Patients should be encouraged to carry their blood glucose testing equipment with them at all times. Physical capabilities to program the pump and monitor its operation are necessary; patients must be able to understand the relationships between components of the treatment plan and their effects on blood glucose levels. Anticipating insulin needs for varying activities increases the likelihood that patients will make the appropriate adjustments in insulin so that blood glucose levels remain in the desired range.

WEARING THE PUMP

The pump must be worn at all times. Removing the pump for >1–2 hours without insulin compensation puts the patient at risk for developing hyperglycemia and ketosis. Patients are frequently concerned about initiating insulin pump therapy because they believe that it will interfere with activities they enjoy. The pump can be worn during most activities, with the exception of contact sports. Pumps are small enough to be worn on a belt, in a pants or shirt pocket, or clipped to underclothing. Various pump clips and cases are available from pump manufacturers. Pumps should not be submerged in hot tubs or worn while scuba diving. Wear the pump close to the body under warm clothing if the temperature is less than 32°F. Consider the possibility that insulin will be exposed to high temperatures during long periods of time outdoors during the summer. A multiple insulin injection regimen might be preferable if the patient will be spending many hours outdoors in extreme temperatures.

During sleep, patients can place their pumps on the bed, under their pillows, or inside of or attached to their clothing. Patients can move relatively unrestricted with longer (31- or 42-inch) infusion set tubing. If the pump is not watertight, it must be removed for showering or placed in a plastic sheath. If engaging in certain water sports, the patient can remove the pump or place the pump in a waterproof holder. Some pumps are watertight for unlimited surface activity and are considered watertight only up to certain water depths and for specified periods of time.

Most patients are concerned about what to do with the insulin pump during sexual activity, but they may not feel comfortable asking about it. If the patient does not bring up the topic, initiate a discussion about sexual activity and pump use. Most couples find that wearing the insulin pump during sexual activity does not interfere with sexual intimacy. If the pump is disconnected during sexual activity, caution the patient to resume insulin pump delivery within an hour or so. After sexual activity, check the tape and infusion set/pod to ensure that the system is intact and secure.

There are alternatives for patients who do not wish to wear their pumps for certain periods of time, including days at the beach, vacations, or an evening out. They can

- if using an infusion set with a disconnect feature, disconnect the pump for up to 1–2 hours depending on the level of activity (leave the needle or cannula in place);
- take injections of rapid- or short-acting insulin before meals and wear the pump at night to provide basal insulin needs; or

Table 7.4 Technical Components of Insulin Pump Therapy

- Pump operation
  - Placement of the battery or batteries
  - Programming the meal bolus and extended or square wave bolus
  - Programming basal rates
  - Preparation and placement of insulin cartridge or syringe and infusion set/pod (priming infusion set)
  - Infusion site selection, rotation, and care
  - Meaning of alarms and how to respond
  - Programming additional basal rates and basal rate programs as needed and temporary basal rate changes
  - Programming additional pump options (e.g., beep or vibrate, bolus calculator, quick bolus options, setting alarms, and history features)
  - Troubleshooting
- Self-monitoring of blood glucose
  - Determining proper technique
  - Confirming accuracy of results
  - Interpreting blood glucose readings
  - Setting blood glucose goals
  - Using linked meter to help calculate required insulin dosages based on personal settings
- Carbohydrate counting and learning relationship between insulin and food
- Using insulin sensitivity/correction factor
- Learning about hypoglycemia and hyperglycemia: symptoms, causes, prevention, treatment
- Learning about unexplained hyperglycemia: causes, prevention, identification, treatment
- Managing sick days
- Dealing with exercise
- Determining options for special occasions
- Deciding on an insulin regimen when insulin pump use is not desired or pump malfunctions
- Determining decision-making strategies for dealing with lifestyle changes

■ use a multiple daily injection regimen of premeal rapid- or short-acting insulin and bedtime Neutral Protamine Hagedorn (NPH) insulin or insulin glargine or insulin detemir until pump therapy is resumed. If insulin glargine or insulin detemir is used, carefully consider when to resume basal insulin delivery because these insulins can have up to a 24-hour duration of action.

The patient may need to increase the premeal dose of short- or rapid-acting insulin by 20–40% when disconnected from the pump. This increase compensates for the missing basal insulin infusion. The dose of long- or intermediate-acting insulin used to provide the overnight insulin requirement should be ~70–80% of the usual total amount of basal insulin taken in 24 hours, or 1.5–2.0 times the amount of basal insulin usually received overnight. If using rapid-acting instead of short-acting insulin with intermediate-acting insulin, patients usually require a dose of NPH in the morning as well as at bedtime because of the short duration of action of the rapid-acting insulin. A small dose of NPH (10–20% of the total daily insulin dose) should be given in the morning in addition to the dose at bedtime (70–80% of the total daily basal dose).

Remind patients that there are some limitations on the timing of insulin and meals while off the pump. More blood glucose monitoring should be performed while using an alternative insulin regimen.

When traveling by air, patients usually do not have problems with airport security while wearing an insulin pump. However, patients may request a letter from their health care provider that documents their need for an insulin pump, pump supplies, and blood glucose monitoring equipment. Because patients cannot carry liquids, such as juice or soda, through airport security, they should carry glucose tablets and then purchase juice or soda after getting through security, if necessary.

Patients who have very tightly controlled blood glucose levels should be aware that changes in altitude have been shown to cause unintended insulin delivery from their pumps. During takeoff, when air pressure decreases, pumps can deliver about one extra unit of insulin on average. During descent, when the pressure is increased, some insulin can be sucked back into the pump, causing the pump to give too little insulin (about 1 unit). Advise the patient to disconnect the pump from the infusion set before takeoff, and to remove air bubbles and reconnect at cruising altitude. Disconnect from the infusion set if there is a sudden drop in cabin pressure. During landing, disconnect the pump. After landing, prime the line with insulin and reconnect the pump.

PATIENT EDUCATION FOR CSII

Appropriate education for insulin pump therapy takes place in three phases (Table 7.3). The first phase occurs before initiating pump therapy. During this period, discuss the advantages and disadvantages of pump therapy, the patient's treatment goals, and the patient's resources to successfully manage insulin pump therapy. Initiate strategies to establish the patient's suitability for insulin pump use, such as a trial of performing and recording four blood glucose tests per day, using a multiple daily insulin regimen with carbohydrate counting, or adding insulin algorithms to an existing insulin regimen before establishing the patient's ISF. With the health care provider's assistance, the patient should choose the pump brand and model and verify insurance coverage and requirements. For example, before approving an insulin pump, some insurance companies require several weeks or months of blood glucose records and an A1c level. A particular pump brand or model may not be covered by the patient's insurance company, necessitating additional paperwork and letters of medical necessity from the health care provider.

After a decision to initiate insulin pump therapy is made, the second phase of education begins. During this period, verify blood glucose–monitoring and meal planning (i.e., carbohydrate counting) skills. This education can be accomplished through a series of outpatient visits with certified diabetes educator(s) (nurse and dietitian). The patient can be given the opportunity to wear the pump for several days, using normal saline to master the technical skills associated with pump therapy and to increase his or her comfort with the idea of wearing a pump. In general, most pump initiations are done on an outpatient basis.

If there is an extenuating circumstance, such as hypoglycemia unawareness or extreme concern regarding nocturnal management, an inpatient stay may be warranted. The inpatient hospitalization could be a 1- to 3-day stay, during which skills learned as an outpatient are verified and refined. Initiate insulin pump therapy on admission to the hospital, and adjust the starting basal rate and insulin bolus doses based on frequent blood glucose monitoring. Remember to instruct the patient to stop intermediate- or long-acting insulin 12–24 hours before initiation of insulin pump therapy and to take injections of short- or rapid-acting insulin every 3–4 hours.

If pump initiation and education are done on an outpatient basis, the patient will need to perform frequent blood glucose monitoring and maintain close contact with the health care team. This contact usually consists of daily phone calls or faxing or emailing blood glucose results, carbohydrate counting, and bolus dose records. Focus on teaching the basic components of insulin pump therapy, including the technical components of the pump (see Table 7.4), the pump's insulin delivery system, carbohydrate counting, monitoring blood glucose, and preventing and treating hypoglycemia and hyperglycemia.

The third phase begins after insulin doses are determined and the patient demonstrates technical competence using the pump. This phase is an intensive period of follow-up lasting 2–6 months, during which the patient masters the skills learned in the second phase and integrates those skills into the usual activities of daily life. Visits with a member of the health care team may take place every 2–3 weeks in addition to weekly phone contact. The patient should keep blood glucose and food records to facilitate learning to quantify food and plan meals and to identify relationships among blood glucose levels, insulin dose and timing, dietary intake, and activity. These records also assist the health care team to modify insulin doses and determine whether the patient understands all of the components of the treatment plan.

When the insulin dosages are fine-tuned to the patient's eating habits and routines and the patient has mastered the components of intensive diabetes management via CSII, ongoing management consists of evaluating the patient's adaptation to pump therapy. Education may focus on teaching the patient to

- use the features of the insulin pump to deal with various situations, such as using the temporary basal rate function during exercise and the extended or combination boluses;
- deal with any insulin pump–related problems, including difficulties in keeping the infusion set/pod securely taped in place, infusion site discomfort, and unexplained hyperglycemia; and
- identify obstacles to achieving treatment goals and develop plans to overcome those obstacles.

SENSOR AUGMENTED PUMP THERAPY

Sensor augmented insulin pump therapy improves glycemic control without increasing the frequency of mild or severe hypoglycemia in people who use continuous glucose monitoring (CGM) on a regular basis. The sensor gives pump users access to continuous glucose readings and alerts/alarms, which can help them better anticipate and manage episodes of hypoglycemia and hyperglycemia.

CGM devices consist of a disposable transcutaneous glucose sensor connected to a transmitter that wirelessly sends glucose readings to the receiver. The sensor is inserted much like an infusion set. The receiver can be a stand-alone unit or can actually be part of the pump, depending on the manufacturer. The screen on the receiver/pump displays the glucose level, along with graphic representations of the glucose levels and arrows that indicate the direction and rate of change in the glucose concentration. Sensors measure interstitial glucose every 5 minutes and transmit readings to the receiver or pump. Sensors require a warm-up period, and require calibration with the patient's blood glucose meter at least twice a day. There are currently 3-day and 7-day sensors.

Sensors alert the patient when glucose levels fall below or rise above individually set glucose limits, and when glucose levels rise or fall rapidly. Trend arrows show the direction and rate of change of the glucose levels. Predictive alerts can be set to warn patients up to 30 minutes before the high or low glucose limits are reached. Depending on the model, up to eight customizable low and high alerts can be set to allow patients to note varying glucose limits throughout the day. The sensors work with data management software that can reveal glucose patterns. One manufacturer's system allows the patient to download integrated pump and sensor data to a secure website that can be accessed by the health care provider in between visits or before visits.

Sensors do not eliminate the need for capillary blood glucose measurements with a meter. The sensor must be calibrated to the patient's blood glucose meter, and sensor readings taken alone are not considered accurate enough to make decisions about insulin dosing at the time of a single observation, but rather, trend analysis may be used prospectively to revise pump settings, and rate of change may be used in real team to cause the user to modify a bolus calculation based on the glucose meter reading and planned carbohydrate intake. There is a physiologic lag time of up to 20 minutes between the blood glucose and interstitial glucose level. This can be problematic when glucose levels are changing rapidly. The FDA has recommended that patients continue to use their blood glucose meters to confirm sensor readings before taking insulin, to confirm a high or low sensor reading, or before making other self-management decisions.

Patient education is an important element of successful sensor-augmented pump therapy. Patients can become frustrated with calibration issues, frequent alarms, and a wide variability of glucose values. Patients can become overwhelmed by the vast amount of data that sensors generate. Instruct patients to calibrate the sensor when glucose levels are not changing rapidly, such as before meals or while in a fasting state. Discuss the patient's schedule to anticipate the best times to insert and calibrate the sensor. Set alarms (threshold glucose and projected glucose alarms) in stages so that the patient can adjust to new stages and master them before moving on to others. Negotiate target ranges that will not frustrate patients by resulting in frequent and annoying alarms. Set a wide target range at first, and narrow the range as patients become more skilled at interpreting and responding to sensor readings and alerts/alarms. Remind patients about the pharmacologic action of insulin so that patients do not administer insulin too often, which can lead to overcorrection of high glucose readings and subsequent hypoglycemia. Close follow-up during the first few weeks of sensor use is essential.

Glucose sensors are especially useful for patients who have hypoglycemia unawareness, severe hypoglycemia or frequent nocturnal hypoglycemia, difficulty achieving target glucose levels, women with gestational diabetes, pregnant women, and children whose parents wish to closely monitor their young children's glucose levels. Cost is another consideration for patients who may benefit from glucose sensors.

THE FUTURE

The improvement in the performance of glucose sensors has renewed interest in developing closed-loop insulin delivery systems that combine a continuous insulin delivery system, a continuous glucose sensor, and an algorithm that links the delivery of insulin to glucose measurements. Different models are being developed and tested as follows: (1) insulin delivery would be suspended or decreased when low glucose levels decrease below a preset threshold and there is no response by the patient to correct the low blood glucose level; this model is intended to minimize hypoglycemia; (2) prediction algorithms would increase or decrease the basal rate to prevent impending hypoglycemia or hyperglycemia; or (3) a fully automated algorithm would restore target blood glucose levels by delivering insulin or changing insulin delivery with minimal user interaction. Challenges involve developing algorithms that will successfully predict glucose values and the rate of change in blood glucose concentration based on individual insulin needs and in response to meals and exercise.

Development of information and communication technology applications for diabetes management are also under consideration. Tasks such as transmitting and exchanging blood glucose and insulin data could be made easier via mobile phones and/or via websites. Cell phones equipped with glucose meters or applications that track blood glucose levels and communicate with health care providers might be a more streamlined way for teenagers and busy professionals to manage their diabetes. Imagine that your glucose sensor could connect to Bluetooth features in your car that can alert you to hypoglycemia and instruct you to pull over and eat a snack. One can imagine a proposed system that integrates a hypoglycemia prediction algorithm with a global position system (GPS) locator and short message service such that the current glucose value and rate of change along with the location of the individual could be communicated to a predefined list of people. If linked to an insulin pump, the system could suspend the pump or decrease the basal rate to prevent the impending event.

Patch pumps that do not require infusion tubing may be configured in a variety of ways in the future. Some may be smaller, flatter, and less expensive. Some may use a separate PDA-like device to program the pump, whereas others may have only basic programming options and no separate programming controller. Others may be more environmentally friendly by making the infusion set and the micropump separate units. The infusion set would be discarded and replaced every 2 to 3 days, but the micropump that snaps onto the infusion set could be designed to last 90 days. Some of the proposed remote controllers could resemble smart phones.

SUMMARY AND CONCLUSION

Insulin pump therapy provides many advantages for patients with diabetes who are seeking improved glycemic control and increased lifestyle flexibility. More physiologic insulin delivery, less variability in insulin absorption, and several technical features that enable patients to modify insulin delivery according to their specific lifestyle requirements make insulin pump therapy an ideal treatment option for individuals seeking greater flexibility and more control over their diabetes self-management. Careful dosing and adjustment of basal and bolus insulin delivery, comprehensive patient education, and ongoing follow-up are essential for successful insulin pump therapy. Sensor augmented insulin pump therapy can assist patients to improve their blood glucose control without increasing the frequency of hypoglycemia. The future is promising as improved technologies are applied to diabetes management.

BIBLIOGRAPHY

Attia N, Jones TW, Holcombe J, Tamborlane WV: Comparison of human regular and lispro insulins after interruption of continuous subcutaneous insulin infusion and in the treatment of acutely decompensated IDDM. *Diabetes Care* 21:817–821, 1998

Bailey T, Ellis S, Garg S, Kaplan R, Jovanovic L, Schwartz S, Zisser H: Improvement in glycemic excursions with a transcutaneous real-time continuous glucose sensor. *Diabetes Care* 29:44–50, 2006

Bergenstal RM, Tamborlane WV, Ahmann A, Buse JB, Dailey G, Davis SN, et al: Effectiveness of sensor-augmented insulin-pump therapy in type 1 diabetes. *N Engl J Med* 363:311–320, 2010

Bode BW, Garg S, Hirsch IB, Hu P, Kolaczynski JW, Lane WS, Santiago OM, Sussman A: Continuous subcutaneous insulin infusion (CSII) of insulin aspart versus multiple daily injection of insulin aspart/insulin glargine in type 1 diabetic patients previously treated with CSII. *Diabetes Care* 28:533–538, 2005

Bode BW, Tamborlane WV, Davidson PC: Insulin pump therapy in the 21st century: strategies for successful use in adults, adolescents, and children with diabetes (Review). *Postgrad Med* 111:69–77, 2002

Corriveau EA, Durso PJ, Kaufman ED, Skipper BJ, Laskaratos LA, Heintzman KB: Effect of Carelink, an internet-based insulin pump monitoring system, on glycemic control in rural and urban children with type 1 diabetes mellitus. *Pediatric Diabetes* 9:360–366, 2008

Dassau E, Cameron F, Lee H, Bequette BW, Zisser H, Jovanovic L, Chase HP, Wilson DM, Buckingham BA, Doyle FJ III: Real-time hypoglycemia prediction suite using continuous glucose monitoring. A safety net for the artificial pancreas. *Diabetes Care* 33:1249–1254, 2010

Dassau E, Jovanovic L, Doyle FJ 3rd, Zisser HC: Enhanced 911/global position system wizard: a telemedicine application for the prevention of severe hypoglycemia—monitor, alert, and locate. *J Diabetes Sci Tech* 3:1501–1506, 2009

Diabetes Control and Complications Trial (DCCT) Research Group: Implementation of treatment protocols in the Diabetes Control and Complications Trial. *Diabetes Care* 18:361–376, 1995

Diabetes Control and Complications Trial (DCCT) Research Group: Hypoglycemia in the Diabetes Control and Complications Trial. *Diabetes* 46:271–286, 1997

Hirsch IB: Algorithms for care in adults using continuous glucose monitoring. *J Diabetes Sci Technol* 1:126–129, 2007

Hirsch IB, Abelseth J, Bode BW, Fischer JS, Kaufman FR, Mastrototaro J, Parkin CG, Wolpert HA, Buckingham BA: Sensor-augmented insulin pump therapy: Results of the first randomized treat-to-target study. *Diabetes Technol Ther* 10:377–383, 2008

Hirsch IB, Armstrong D, Bergenstal RM, Buckingham B, Childs BP, Clarke WL, Peters A, Wolpert H: Clinical application of emerging sensor technologies in diabetes management: Consensus guidelines for continuous glucose monitoring (CGM). *Diabetes Technology & Therapeutics* 10:232–246, 2008

Juvenile Diabetes Research Foundation Continuous Glucose Monitoring Study Group: Continuous glucose monitoring and intensive treatment of type 1 diabetes. *NEJM* 359:1464–1476, 2008

Juvenile Diabetes Research Foundation Continuous Glucose Monitoring Study Group: The effect of continuous glucose monitoring in well-controlled type 1 diabetes. *Diabetes Care* 32:1378–1383, 2009

Keen H, Pickup J: Continuous subcutaneous insulin infusion at 25 years. *Diabetes Care* 25:593–598, 2002

King BR, Goss PW, Paterson MA, Crock PA, Anderson DG: Changes in altitude cause unintended insulin delivery from insulin pumps: Mechanisms and implications. *Diabetes Care* 34:1932–1933, 2011

Kovatchev B, Cobelli C, Renard E, Anderson S, Breton M, Patek S, Clarke W, Bruttomesso D, Maran A, Costa S, Avogaro A, Dalla Mann C, Facchinetti A, Magni L, DeNicolao G, Place J, Farret A: Multinational study of subcutaneous model-predictive closed-loop control in type 1 diabetes mellitus: Summary of the results. *J Diabetes Sci Tech* 4:1374–1381, 2010

Lenhard MJ, Reeves GD: Continuous subcutaneous insulin infusion: a comprehensive review of insulin pump therapy. *Arch Intern Med* 161:2293–2300, 2001

Phillip M, Battelino T, Rodriguez H, Danne T, Kaufman F: Use of insulin pump therapy in the pediatric age group: consensus statement from the European Society for Paediatric Endocrinology, the Lawson Wilkins Pediatric Endocrine Society, and the International Society for Pediatric and Adolescent Diabetes, endorsed by the American Diabetes Association and the European Association for the Study of Diabetes. *Diabetes Care* 30:1653–1662, 2007

Pickup J, Keen H: Continuous subcutaneous insulin infusion at 25 years: evidence base for the expanding use of insulin pump therapy in type 1 diabetes (Review). *Diabetes Care* 25:593–598, 2002

Walsh J, Roberts R: *Pumping Insulin*. 4th ed. San Diego, CA, Torrey Pines Press, 2007

Wang Y, Dassau E, Zisser H, Jovanovic L, Doyle F III: Automatic bolus and adaptive basal algorithm for the artificial pancreative β-cell. *Diabetes Technol Ther* 12:879–887, 2010

Monitoring

Highlights
Monitoring

- Regular monitoring is an essential component of any diabetes regimen. During intensive diabetes management, monitoring is even more important and must be done more frequently than during conventional treatment.

- Monitoring during intensive diabetes management includes self-monitoring of blood glucose (SMBG) as well as urine and blood ketone monitoring and also continuous glucose monitoring (CGM).

- Monitoring of blood glucose during symptoms of hypoglycemia is strongly recommended, as is monitoring before driving an automobile.

- Monitoring of metabolic control by the health care team at each visit should include
  - glycated hemoglobin (A1c) – estimated average glucose,
  - review of blood glucose records, and
  - assessment of growth, weight, and blood pressure.

- Converting A1c measurements into an estimated average glucose value helps "translate" the A1c into a number patients can understand, and makes treatment goals more tangible.

- Real-time continuous glucose monitoring (RT-CGM) is a promising new technology that reduces the risk for hypoglycemia associated with intensification of glucose control.

- Monitoring the development and progression of long-term complications of diabetes should be performed at least as often as proposed by the American Diabetes Association in its Standards of Medical Care (see Monitoring for Long-Term Complications).

Monitoring

Regular monitoring is an essential component of any diabetes management regimen. In intensive diabetes management, monitoring is even more important and must be done more frequently than in conventional treatment regimens. This is true for both the medical monitoring performed by the health care team and the day-to-day monitoring required by the patient. Patient monitoring includes self-monitoring of blood glucose (SMBG), ketone monitoring, and continuous glucose monitoring (CGM). Monitoring by health care providers includes regular determination of glycated hemoglobin (A1c), careful assessment of growth and development (in both children and adolescents) and weight (in adults), careful review of hypoglycemia episodes and related complications, review of ketone monitoring and sick-day management, and monitoring for the presence of long-term diabetes complications.

MONITORING BY THE PATIENT

All patients using an intensive diabetes management program are expected to perform monitoring on a daily basis at home, work, school, or wherever they may be. This includes SMBG, ketone testing, and careful record keeping of the results.

BLOOD GLUCOSE

When implementing an intensive diabetes management regimen, patients often will perform SMBG four to six times a day. An inability or unwillingness to perform SMBG should be considered a contraindication to implementing intensive diabetes therapy. The expectation should be for at least three to four SMBG determinations a day. An intensive diabetes management regimen rarely can be optimally successful without monitoring blood glucose at least four times a day, and should not be recommended if the patient performs fewer than three blood glucose determinations a day.

The four essential SMBG determinations for successful implementation of an intensive diabetes management regimen must be performed before each meal and before bedtime. Premeal measurements are needed to determine the dose of insulin and/or meal or activity alterations required to achieve the target glucose level over the next few hours. They also are used to determine patterns of glycemia over time that will guide adjustment of the regimen. It is best to observe these patterns over periods of at least 3–5 days before making an overall change in the regimen. The bedtime blood glucose measurement is essential to assess the adequacy of the dinnertime dose of insulin and is also a key safety component in preventing nocturnal hypoglycemia. The morning value is used to assess the adequacy of overnight glycemic control.

Recent reports stress the importance of postprandial glycemia to achieve and maintain target A1c values and prevent micro- and macrovascular disease complications. Two to three hour postprandial glucose determinations are essential to determine optimal meal insulin doses. After the appropriate meal insulin doses have been determined, postprandial monitoring for each meal remains important and should be performed at least once a week to verify the correct bolus or meal insulin doses.

In addition to these four blood glucose determinations, monitoring should include a periodic blood glucose measurement between 2:00 and 4:00 a.m. to detect unrecognized nocturnal hypoglycemia, especially for patients in whom the target blood glucose range is near the nondiabetic range or for patients in whom nocturnal or severe hypoglycemia or hypoglycemia unawareness has been a problem. Nocturnal monitoring may need to be performed more often than once a week during periods when the basal insulin dose is being adjusted.

Monitoring blood glucose when symptoms of hypoglycemia occur is strongly recommended. Because hypoglycemia can occur with few or no early warning symptoms (hypoglycemia unawareness) and autonomic (adrenergic) symptoms can occur in the absence of hypoglycemia, it is recommended that patient's confirm biochemical hypoglycemia, and by measuring the blood glucose level when symptoms occur.

Because some patients' driving ability may be impaired at blood glucose levels higher than those that usually trigger easily recognizable hypoglycemia symptoms (especially in patients with hypoglycemia unawareness and those using intensive diabetes therapy), it is strongly recommended that blood glucose be monitored before driving.

KETONE MONITORING

Monitoring for the presence of ketones is an essential component of diabetes care. There are certain situations in which ketone monitoring is necessary for the safe implementation of diabetes therapy, regardless of the type of therapy used (Table 8.1).

Ketone monitoring can be done using strips that measure urine ketones (acetoacetate and acetone) or with a meter that measures blood beta-hydroxybutyrate concentration. This device is similar to other SMBG meters and can also measure blood glucose levels using a different strip in the same meter. The advantages of urine-monitoring strips are the ease of sample collection under most circumstances and their low cost. Measurement of blood ketones offers the special advantage in young children who may not cooperate during urine ketone testing, especially during illness. Additionally, during a gastrointestinal illness, modest dehydration may result in concentrated urine, causing the urine ketone determination to indicate severe ketonuria although the blood ketone value is not markedly elevated. Under these circumstances, measurement of blood ketone levels may prevent a trip to the emergency room. Blood ketone determination is significantly more expensive than urine ketone determination, but in some circumstances may be cost-effective.

Table 8.1 Patient Monitoring During Intensive Diabetes Management

- Self-monitoring of blood glucose
  - Before each meal
  - At bedtime
  - Between 2:00 and 4:00 a.m. at least weekly
  - When symptoms of hypoglycemia occur
  - Before driving
- Ketone monitoring
  - During any illness
  - During unexpected or persistent hyperglycemia
  - During times of weight loss (intentional or unexpected)
  - Daily during pregnancy
- Record keeping

Blood or urine ketones should be checked whenever the blood glucose level is unexpectedly or repeatedly >250–300 mg/dl (>13.8–16.7 mmol/l). The same is true during intercurrent illness, especially a gastrointestinal illness, regardless of the blood glucose concentration. Illness can trigger diabetic ketoacidosis; therefore, which rapid identification and intervention can prevent severe illness and possible hospitalization. In addition, ketosis itself can cause abdominal pain and vomiting.

For patients using an insulin pump, ketones should be measured whenever there is "unexplained" hyperglycemia. In this setting, the presence of ketonuria and/or ketonemia may indicate failure of the insulin delivery system. Finally, it is recommended that urinary ketones be monitored daily in women who are pregnant.

RECORD KEEPING

Carefully organized recording of SMBG results should be considered an essential component of intensive diabetes management. Many blood glucose meters have a memory that stores blood glucose values together with the date and time of day, and data can be downloaded to a computer. In addition, maintenance of a written log can be important. Unless patients are able to download the results and review them every few days, they would not be able to examine their records in a way that enables them to look for patterns over 3–5 days and then make necessary adjustments in their regimen.

It is useful to record blood glucose values in a format that enables all the results for a given day to be arrayed across a single row and with the results for the same time of day over many days to line up in columns. Ideally, several days should be logged on a single page. This format enables the patient and health care provider to quickly scan the log. Blood glucose values for any given day are reviewed by looking across a single row. All the results for a given time of day (e.g., prelunch) are reviewed by looking down a single column. This format is the most effective for identifying patterns and trends.

It is also helpful if the log has spaces for recording insulin doses, hypoglycemia episodes, and additional notes and comments. Some highly conscientious and motivated patients will highlight their blood glucose log with one color for values below the target and with another color for values above the target. Although this approach is not essential, it can be helpful to identify trends. For example, if a quick glance at the records were to show several yellow-highlighted values (when the patient used yellow to indicate a low blood glucose level), then it is easy to detect when a lower insulin dose may be needed.

Many blood glucose meters now have the capability to download data into a computerized database for analysis and long-term storage. Use of such computerized databases is not essential to the successful implementation of diabetes care; however, some health care providers find it helpful to observe SMBG results in one of the various graphic, tabular, or text formats provided by these computer software systems. Reviewing the results on the computer screen with the patient at the time of a visit can be helpful and educational in some settings.

Many blood glucose meters also now have internal data analysis capability and can display blood glucose averages, modal day graphs, and other helpful patterns for patient. Many meters connect to or are easily downloaded to home computers or handheld computer devices. These devices allow patients to more easily detect trends in blood glucose values and identify when insulin dose changes are needed.

MONITORING BY THE HEALTH CARE TEAM

Overall metabolic control in people with diabetes is assessed primarily by four factors:

- Average overall blood glucose and A1c levels
- Frequency and severity of hypoglycemia
- Adequacy of growth, weight gain, and physical development in children and weight in adults
- Plasma lipid levels

At the outset of intensive diabetes management, after daily to weekly office visits when the program is being implemented and adjusted, the patient will require scheduled visits to assess the success of the program (Table 8.2).

It is common practice to assess a patient's glycemic control and general health status quarterly. This schedule usually is sufficient for the patient using intensive diabetes management after the initial phase of stabilization. At each visit,

- measure A1c;
- check accuracy of blood glucose–monitoring;
- review blood glucose data;
- study problems with hypoglycemia;
- identify and discuss any barriers to intensive diabetes management;
- discuss issues of diet;
- note body weight, blood pressure, and growth and physical development in children; and
- examine sites of insulin administration.

Table 8.2 Monitoring Metabolic Control

- Routinely determine A1c (estimated average glucose)
- Review SMBG results carefully at every visit, as well as between visits (if necessary)
- Review the frequency, severity, recognition, and treatment of hypoglycemia
- Assess growth, weight gain, and physical development in children and adolescents and weight in adults
- Take a careful history related to the management of sick days and occurrence of keto-acidosis
- Review issues of diet, including weight, and any difficulties in adherence to the overall management plan
- Monitor blood lipids annually

A1C – ESTIMATED AVERAGE GLUCOSE

The A1c test reflects mean glycemia over the preceding 2–3 months, and is an essential component of diabetes management. The A1c should be measured at least twice a year in patients who are meeting treatment goals, and quarterly in patients whose therapy has changed or who are not at goal. Monthly A1c measurments may be useful during periods of changing diabetes regimens. Converting A1c measurements into an estimated average glucose value helps "translate" the A1c into a number that patients can understand more readily, and may make treatment goals more tangible (Table 8.3). However, individual variations in the rate of hemoglobin glycation can contribute to inaccuracy in estimating the average glucose from A1c levels, and it is important for clinicians to inform patients about this uncertainty.

A1c can be measured by several different methods. In recent years the International Federation of Clinical Chemistry and Laboratory Medicine (IFCC) has developed a new method that specifically measures the concentration of one molecular species of A1c. This new IFCC method allows for

Table 8.3 Correlation between A1c Level and Estimated Average Glucose Level

	Glucose Level	
A1c (%)	mg/dl (95% CIs)	mmol/l
6	126 (100–152)	7.0 (5.5–8.5)
7	154 (123–185)	8.6 (6.8–10.3)
8	183 (147–217)	10.2 (8.1–12.1)
9	212 (170–249)	11.8 (9.4–13.9)
10	240 (193–282)	13.4 (10.7–15.7)
11	269 (217–314)	14.9 (12.0–17.5)
12	298 (240–347)	16.5 (13.3–19.3)

worldwide standardization of A1c measurements performed using different methodologies. Adoption of this new reference standard will facilitate direct comparison of A1c measurements from different laboratories and will ensure the accuracy of the A1c-derived average glucose measurements used for clinical care.

Although the A1c level gives reliable information about the average blood glucose level over the preceding 6–12 weeks, it still is essential for the health care provider to review the blood glucose record carefully at each visit and, when appropriate, between visits as well. The use of the telephone, fax. or email is helpful for between visits. This review should keep in mind the individualized goals for blood glucose level and should include an overall inspection of the blood glucose values since the last visit, as well as an examination for patterns of hyper- and hypoglycemia. Identification of patterns should trigger a change in regimen. If there is considerable discrepancy between the A1c result and the recorded SMBG values, the reason for this discrepancy should be sought.

REAL-TIME CONTINUOUS GLUCOSE MONITORING

In the past few years, several real-time CGM (RT-CGM) devices (Abbott's FreeStyle Navigator®, DexCom's SEVEN®, Medtronic's Guardian®, and Paradigm® systems) have received regulatory approval for use by ambulatory patients with diabetes. This technology measures the interstitial glucose concentration every few minutes and provides the patient with detailed information on glucose patterns and trends, with alarms that are triggered by both hyper- and hypoglycemia. Current RT-CGM devices approved for long-term clinical use have transcutaneous sensors that need to be replaced every 3–7 days. These devices are generally less accurate than current finger-stick capillary blood glucose meters; however, this limitation is offset by the additional information about the rate and direction of changes in the glucose level. Recent trial data indicate that use of RT-CGM by patients with type 1 diabetes can lead to a reduction in A1c *without* an associated increase in hypoglycemia. These findings are in contrast to intervention studies (such as the Diabetes Control and Complications Trial [DCCT]) in which patients used intermittent capillary glucose monitoring to guide diabetes self-management.

To use this technology safely and effectively, patients need to have advanced diabetes self-management skills and must understand several key concepts (including physiologic lag). Currently available CGM devices measure glucose in the interstitial fluid in the subcutaneous tissue, whereas glucose meters measure capillary blood glucose obtained by finger stick. When the glucose concentration is changing, there is a physiologic lag in the equilibration of glucose between these two compartments. This lag has important implications for accuracy of continuous glucose sensors and the use of RT-CGM in diabetes self-management. RT-CGM does not eliminate the need for finger-stick capillary blood glucose measurements. These measurements are required to calibrate the sensor and confirm glucose readings prior to an insulin bolus. The alarms for hypo- and hyperglycemia are an important feature of RT-CGM devices. To ensure that the patient derives maximum benefit from use of the alarms, the alarm thresholds must be individualized. If alarm thresholds are set at the "ideal" level (e.g., low = 90 mg/dl, high = 180 mg/dl), the patient will be warned of most low and high glucose values; however, there will also be frequent false alarms with increased risk for "alarm burnout" and a related tendency to ignore the alarms. Conversely, if alarm thresholds are set more widely (e.g., low = 60 mg/dl, high = 240 mg/dl), there will be few false alarms and less risk for "alarm burnout"; however, the patient will not be warned about all low and high glucose values.

MONITORING FOR LONG-TERM COMPLICATIONS

The long-term complications of diabetes include retinopathy and cataracts; renal insufficiency and hypertension; autonomic and peripheral neuropathy; and macrovascular disease manifested by myocardial infarction, stroke, and peripheral vascular disease. Although improved glycemic control, with intensive diabetes therapy, delays the onset and slows the progression of retinopathy, nephropathy, and neuropathy and improves the risk factor profile related to macrovascular disease, complications of diabetes have not yet been eliminated. Therefore, monitoring for their presence and appropriate intervention or referral to appropriate specialists are required (Table 8.4).

RETINAL EXAMINATIONS

A comprehensive examination by an optometrist or ophthalmologist is recommended for all patients with type 2 diabetes at the time of diagnosis, for all patients with type 1 diabetes within 5 years after diagnosis, and for any patient with diabetes who has visual symptoms or abnormalities. Subsequent examinations should be repeated at least annually, or more frequently if advanced retinopathy is noted. Women who are planning pregnancy or who are pregnant should also have a comprehensive eye examination, and require ophthalmologic follow-up throughout pregnancy.

Retinopathy may initially worsen during the first months of intensive diabetes management. This worsening is more often reported in patients who have poor glycemic control and more advanced retinopathy prior to the initiation of intensive therapy. In the DCCT, retinopathy progression was greater in the intensively treated cohort at the end of the first year. By the end of the second year, this difference was not significant, and thereafter the intensively treated cohort had a lower rate of retinopathy progression. Therefore, anyone undertaking intensive management should have a retinal examination before beginning intensive management, and should discuss the plans for intensive management with his or her eye care professional, especially if metabolic control has been poor.

LIPID SCREENING

Lipid abnormalities play an important role in macrovascular disease. In recognition of this, diabetes is regarded as a risk factor for cardiovascular events equivalent to a previous cardiac event. A fasting lipid profile should be measured every year in patients whose values fall within acceptable risk levels. The profile should

Table 8.4 Monitoring for Long-Term Complications

- Comprehensive annual dilated eye and visual examination, beginning
  - when diagnosed with type 2 diabetes
  - duration of type 1 diabetes of 3–5 years (and ≥10 years old)
  - age >30 years, regardless of duration
  - any visual symptoms/abnormalities
- Monitor blood lipids annually
- Careful examination of the feet (sensation, pulses, reflexes) at each visit
- Careful assessment of blood pressure at each visit
- Annual determination of urinary albumin after diabetes duration of 3–5 years (patients with type 1 diabetes); children ≥10 years old; at diagnosis and annually thereafter (patients with type 2 diabetes)
- Monitor serum creatinine annually for determination of estimated glomerular filtration rate (eGFR) in all adults regardless of urine microalbumin excretion

be assessed more often in patients with abnormal lipid values or inadequate blood glucose control. Abnormal lipid values should trigger intervention, including dietary and exercise counseling, attempts to achieve better glycemic control, and lipid-lowering medication, as indicated. Guidelines for low-density lipoprotein (LDL) levels are shown in Table 8.5.

BLOOD PRESSURE

Blood pressure should be measured at each visit. If it is elevated, repeated measures should be taken to confirm the presence of hypertension, and antihypertensive therapy should be implemented (Table 8.6). Most epidemiological studies have suggested that risk caused by elevated blood pressure is a continuous function; therefore, blood pressure cutoff levels are arbitrary. However, recent intervention studies in patients with type 2 diabetes suggest that lowering the systolic blood pressure from low 130s to <120 mmHg does not reduce cardiac events or death, although a significant reduction in stroke was seen. Blood pressure goals for most patients with type 1 diabetes should be <130 mmHg for systolic and <80 mmHg for diastolic blood pressure. If treatment to this goal is achieved and well tolerated, further lowering may be beneficial. In children, blood pressure should be decreased to the corresponding age, gender, and height adjusted 90th percentile values.

URINARY ALBUMIN SCREENING

Measurement of urinary albumin excretion should be performed annually in all individuals ≥10 years old with type 1 diabetes duration of at least 3–5 years. Because of the difficulty in precisely dating the onset of type 2 diabetes, such screening should begin at the time of diagnosis. Screening for microalbuminuria can be performed by measuring the albumin-to-creatinine ratio in a random, spot urine collection. Screen-

Table 8.5 Glycemic, Blood Pressure, and Lipid Goals or Ideal Values (for Nonpregnant Adults)

A1c	<7%*
Blood pressure	<130/80 mmHg†
Lipids	
LDL	<100 mg/dl (<2.6 mmol/l)‡

*More or less stringent glycemic goals may be appropriate for individual patients. Goals should be individualized based on duration of diabetes, age/life expectancy, comorbid conditions, known CVD or advancedmicrovascular complications, hypoglycemia unawareness, individual and patient considerations.

†Based on patient characteristics and response to therapy, higher or lower SBP targets may be appropriate.

‡In individuals with overt CVD, a lower LDL cholesterol goal of 70 mg/dL (1.8 mmol/L), using a high dose of a statin, is an option

ing may be confounded by orthostatic proteinuria; therefore, abnormal results should be repeated on first morning urine specimens.

FOOT EXAMINATIONS

At each visit, carefully examined the feet with the patient's socks and shoes removed. The examination should include inspection to assess hygiene and to determine the presence of any ulcers or infection. The assessment also should include a careful history to ascertain the presence of numbness, paresthesiae (tingling), or weakness. Pulses should be palpated, and reflexes and sensation should be checked.

BIBLIOGRAPHY

American Diabetes Association: Preventive foot care in people with diabetes (Position Statement). *Diabetes Care* 27 (Suppl. 1):S63–S64, 2004

American Diabetes Association: Standards of medical care in Diabetes—2012. *Diabetes Care* 35 (Suppl. 1):S11–S63, 2012

American Diabetes Association, European Association for the Study of Diabetes, International Federation of Clinical Chemistry and Laboratory Medicine, and the International Diabetes Federation: Consensus statement on the worldwide standardization of hemoglobin A1C measurement. *Diabetes Care* 30:2399–2400, 2007

Cox D, Gonder-Frederick L, Polonsky W, Schlundt D, Julian D, Clarke W: A multicenter evaluation of blood glucose awareness training II. *Diabetes Care* 18:523–528, 1995

Cryer PE, Shamoon H: Hypoglycemia in diabetes. *Diabetes Care* 26:1902–1912, 2003

Fong DS, Aiello LP, Ferris FL III, Klein R: Diabetic retinopathy. *Diabetes Care* 27:2540–2553, 2004

Juvenile Diabetes Research Foundation Continuous Glucose Monitoring Study Group, Tamborlane WV, Beck RW, Bode BW, Buckingham B, Chase HP, Clemons R, Fiallo-Scharer R, Fox LA, Gilliam LK, Hirsch IB, Huang ES, Kollman C, Kowalski AJ, Laffel L, Lawrence JM, Lee J, Mauras N, O'Grady M, Ruedy KJ, Tansey M, Tsalikian E, Weinzimer S, Wilson DM, Wolpert H, Wysocki T, Xing D: Continuous glucose monitoring and intensive treatment of type 1 diabetes. *N Engl J Med* 359:1464–1476, 2008

Nathan DM, Kuenen J, Borg R, Zheng H, Schoenfeld D, Heine R: Translating the A1c assay into estimated average glucose values. *Diabetes Care* 31:1–6, 2008

Wilson DM, Xing D, Cheng J, Beck RW, Hirsch I, Kollman C, Laffel L, Lawrence JM, Mauras N, Ruedy K, Tsalikian E, Wolpert H: Juvenile Diabetes Research Foundation Continuous Glucose Monitoring Study Group: Persistence of individual variations in glycated hemoglobin. *Diabetes Care* 34:1315–1317, 2011

Wolpert H: The nuts and bolts of achieving end points with real-time continuous glucose monitoring. *Diabetes Care* 31 (Suppl. 2):S146–S149, 2008

Nutrition Management

Highlights
Nutrition Management

- Medical nutrition therapy (MNT) is integral to the implementation of all intensified forms of diabetes care.

- The primary goals of MNT are to promote metabolic control (including near-normal blood glucose and lipid levels), blood pressure control, and appropriate weight management. The nutrition plan must also prevent, or at least slow, the development of long-term diabetes complications, address individual nutrition needs (taking into account personal preferences and willingness to change), and promote pleasurable eating.

- MNT is often the most challenging aspect of diabetes management, leading to the recommendation that every person with diabetes regularly consult a registered dietitian knowledgeable about diabetes for development and periodic reevaluation of a personalized meal plan. Outcome studies demonstrate that MNT provided by registered dietitians can result in a 1–2% decrease in glycated hemoglobin (A1c).

- Target nutrition recommendations:
  - Urge development of a personalized plan based on an individual assessment
  - Emphasize total carbohydrate intake as the primary nutrition factor affecting postprandial blood glucose levels, but also consider the type of carbohydrate ingested and the fat content of the meal
  - Emphasize the role of weight loss in type 2 diabetes as a strategy for decreasing insulin resistance and achieving glycemic and metabolic control

- In type 1 diabetes, the meal plan should be based on the patient's usual intake with respect to calories, food selection, and meal timing. The insulin regimen should be fitted to the meal plan and adjusted based on the results of glucose monitoring.

- In type 2 diabetes, the dietitian should review the patient's usual intake and advise the patient to distribute calories and carbohydrates throughout the day, avoiding large concentrations at any one time. If the patient is overweight, a moderate calorie restriction (250–500 kcal/day) should be recommended, in concert with advice regarding physical activity and other behavioral or lifestyle modifications, as needed.

- Carbohydrate counting is a meal-planning approach well-suited to intensive diabetes management because it allows matching of meal-time insulin delivery to carbohydrate-related insulin requirement.

- Glucose monitoring is an essential component of all approaches to intensified diabetes management. The joint evaluation of food and glucose records is a powerful tool for glucose control, and allows fine-tuning of both nutrition and medication treatment plans.
- Hypoglycemia is a significant risk of intensive management. Nutrition factors often play a role in the cause and prevention of hypoglycemia.
- Greater precision in glucose control can be promoted through calibrated treatment of hypoglycemia, taking into account both the patient's dose response to oral glucose and the current and target glucose values.
- Weight gain may accompany intensive management when significant improvement in glucose control is achieved and is related to reduction of glycosuria and consumption of extra calories to treat more frequent hypoglycemia. Strategies to prevent weight gain include reducing calories at the outset of intensive management, increasing physical activity, and rigorous MNT.

Nutrition Management

Medical nutrition therapy (MNT) is integral to the successful implementation of all forms of diabetes care. For intensive diabetes management, nutrition aspects of the diabetes care plan are especially important. Patients who use physiological insulin regimens and frequent capillary blood glucose and/or continuous glucose monitoring (CGM) to maintain tight glucose control must apply sophisticated nutrition management skills to fully realize the potential of their intensive management plan. As demonstrated in the Diabetes Control and Complications Trial (DCCT), extensive, individualized nutrition training and problem solving are required to support effective intensive management in patients with type 1 diabetes.

When considering intensifying the management of patients with type 2 diabetes, it is important to note that most patients with type 2 diabetes receive little or no nutrition counseling before starting insulin therapy. Insulin initiation appears to be the most common factor that triggers primary care physicians to refer patients with type 2 diabetes for nutrition management. Those patients who manage their diabetes with lifestyle modification and/or oral hypoglycemic agents or for whom nutrition is the primary or sole treatment modality are least likely to receive assistance with the nutrition component of their management. Clearly, extending MNT to this population would, in itself, represent a major "intensification" of their care.

GOALS OF MNT

The overall goal of MNT in diabetes is to promote metabolic control. Included in this general objective are several specific targets (Table 9.1). To achieve these goals, dietitians and other health care professionals must educate people with diabetes to manage their nutrition intake in respect to a variety of individual factors, which include medication, exercise, illness and other stressors, and lifestyle considerations (e.g., work or school schedules; personal preferences; motivation; and economic, cultural, and religious concerns).

Consistent management and/or modification of food intake are often the most complex and challenging aspects of diabetes care. The complexity of these tasks is due to many factors (Table 9.2) and is the reason for the recommendation that every person with prediabetes or diabetes should consult a registered dietitian (RD), preferably one familiar with the components of diabetes MNT, to obtain an individualized nutrition plan. Because of the interaction of nutrition intake

Table 9.1 Goals of MNT Applicable to All Individuals with Diabetes

- Achieve and maintain:
  - Blood glucose levels in the normal range or as close to normal as is safely possible
  - Blood lipid and lipoprotein profile that reduces the risk for cardiovascular and peripheral vascular disease
  - Blood pressure levels in the normal range or as close to normal as is safely possible
- Prevent (or at least slow) the rate of development of the chronic complications of diabetes by modifying nutrient intake and lifestyle
- Address individual nutrition needs, taking into account personal and cultural preferences and willingness to change
- Maintain the pleasure of eating by only limiting food choices when indicated by scientific evidence

with medication and exercise in determining blood glucose levels, nutrition care must also be fully integrated with other aspects of diabetes management to be effective. This is best accomplished through a team approach; However, at a minimum, successful MNT requires open communication between the dietitian and other care providers. Furthermore, patients who are using intensified regimens, benefit from a series of encounters dedicated to nutrition education and problem solving to help develop the sophisticated skills required for successful management. Regular review and adjustment of the nutrition plan are also needed for optimal results.

TARGET NUTRITION RECOMMENDATIONS

The current nutrition principles and recommendations for diabetes, as formulated by the American Diabetes Association, focus on lifestyle goals and strategies for both the prevention and treatment of diabetes (Table 9.3).

Table 9.2 Factors That Contribute to the Complexity of Nutrition Care

- Interaction of diabetes MNT with coexisting pathology (e.g., abnormal lipids, elevated blood pressure, and other health problems)
- Need to integrate MNT into the other components of the diabetes treatment regimen
- Need for advanced problem-solving skills to permit self-management
- Need for stepwise training to progressively build requisite knowledge and skills
- Inherent difficulty in modifying lifelong food behaviors and preferences
- Dynamic nature of both diabetes and life circumstances that demands periodic and creative modification of the food plan to address changing and often unpredictable factors
- Need to meet all of the above challenges while preserving the patient's autonomy and quality of life

Table 9.3 Target Nutrition Recommendations for All People with Diabetes

Carbohydrate

- A dietary pattern that includes carbohydrate from fruits, vegetables, whole grains, legumes, and low-fat milk is encouraged for good health.
- Monitoring carbohydrate, whether by carbohydrate counting, choices, or experience-based estimation, is a key strategy in achieving glycemic control.
- The use of the glycemic index and glycemic load may modestly improve glycemic control (at least when compared to considering total carbohydrate alone).
- Sucrose-containing foods can be substituted for other carbohydrates in the meal plan or, if added to the meal plan, covered with insulin or other glucose-lowering medications. Care should be taken to avoid excess energy intake.
- Sugar alcohols and nonnutritive sweeteners are safe when consumed within the daily intake levels established by the U.S. Food and Drug Administration.
- People with diabetes are encouraged to consume a variety of fiber-containing foods. There is no evidence, however, to recommend a higher fiber intake for people with diabetes than for the general population.

Protein

- For individuals with diabetes and normal renal function, there is insufficient evidence to suggest that usual protein intake (15–20% of energy) should be modified.
- In individuals with type 2 diabetes, ingested protein can increase insulin response without increasing plasma glucose concentrations. Therefore, protein should not be used to treat acute hypoglycemia or prevent nighttime hypoglycemia.
- High protein diets are not recommended as a method for weight loss.
- The long-term effects of protein intake >20% of calories on diabetes management are unknown. Although such diets may produce short-term weight loss and improve glycemia, it has not been established that these benefits are maintained, and long-term effects on kidney function for persons with diabetes are unknown.

Fat

- Saturated fat intake should be <7% of calories.
- Reducing intake of trans fat lowers LDL cholesterol and increases HDL cholesterol. therefore, intake of trans fats should be minimized.
- Limit dietary cholesterol to <200 mg/dl.
- Two or more servings of fish per week (with the exception of commercially fried fish filets) provide polyunsaturated fatty acids and are recommended.

Macronutrients

- The best mix of carbohydrate, protein, and fat may be adjusted to meet the metabolic goals and individual preferences of the person with diabetes.

Micronutrients

- There is no clear evidence of benefit from vitamin or mineral supplementation, in people with diabetes (compared with the general population) who do not have underlying deficiencies.
- Individualized meal planning should include optimization of food choices to meet recommended daily allowance (RDA)/dietary reference intake (DRI) for all micronutrients.

Table 9.3 (*continued*)

- Routine supplementation with antioxidants, such as vitamins E and C and carotene, is not advised because of lack of evidence of efficacy and concern related to long-term safety. B12 deficiency can also occur.
- Benefit from chromium supplementation in individuals with diabetes or obesity has not been clearly demonstrated and, therefore, cannot be recommended.

Alcohol

- If adults with diabetes choose to consume alcohol, daily intake should be limited to a moderate amount (one drink per day or less for adult women and two drinks per day or less for adult men). One drink is defined as a 12-oz beer, 5 oz of wine, or 1.5 oz of ~80 proof spirits.
- To reduce the risk of nocturnal hypoglycemia in individuals using insulin or insulin secretagogues, alcohol should be consumed with food.
- In individuals with diabetes, moderate consumption of alcohol alone has no acute effect on glucose and insulin concentrations, but when combined with carbohydrate-containing beverage (mixed drinks), it may raise blood glucose.

A personalized nutrition prescription should be based on individual assessment and should consider treatment goals and lifestyle changes the patient is willing and able to make. Clinical outcomes should be monitored and, if necessary, the nutrition prescription should be modified. This method has replaced specific guidelines for one "standard" diet or meal-planning method for all people with diabetes.

The recommendations acknowledge scientific evidence that sucrose and other simple sugars do not inherently impair diabetes control, opening the way for the inclusion of many traditionally "forbidden" foods in diabetes meal plans.

Modest weight loss decreases insulin resistance in individuals with diabetes who are overweight or obese. However, the overarching goal for people with diabetes is to achieve blood glucose, blood pressure, and blood lipid levels in the normal range, or as close to normal as is safely possible, whether by weight loss or other means.

Standardized diets and simplistic advice to "avoid sugar" and "lose weight," which have too often comprised the totality of nutrition advice, are clearly inadequate. The current guidelines are compatible with a shift to more intensified programs of management for all people with diabetes. A flow chart describing the major steps in the design and implementation of meal plans consistent with the current recommendations is shown in Fig. 9.1.

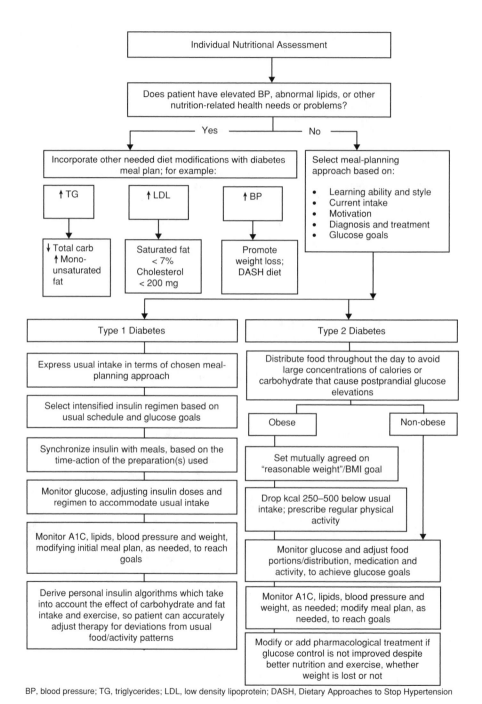

BP, blood pressure; TG, triglycerides; LDL, low density lipoprotein; DASH, Dietary Approaches to Stop Hypertension

Figure 9.1 Nutrition management flow chart (updated).

Table 9.4 Integrating Recommendations Into the Nutrition Care Process

Implementation of MNT:

- Upon diagnosis or first referral to a dietitian, 3–4 encounters lasting 45–90 minutes are recommended within 3–6 months.
- The dietitian should then determine whether additional MNT encounters are needed.
- At least 1 follow-up encounter annually is recommended to reinforce education and/or lifestyle changes, evaluate/monitor outcomes, and determine any need for change in MNT or medications. Dietitian should determine if additional MNT encounters are needed throughout the year.

Nutrition Assessment

- Client History: Medication and supplement history, past medical history, family hisotry, and social history.
- Food/Nutrition History: Food intake (composition, carbohydrate, adequacy, meal/snack patterns, environmental cues to eating, tolerance, currents diets or food modifications); nutrition health awareness and management (knowledge and beliefs about nutrition recommendations, self-monitoring/management practices, prior education); physical activity and exercise (functional status, activity patterns, sedentary time, exercise intensity, frequency, and duration); and food availability (food planning, purchasing, preparation abilities and limitations, food safety, food program utilization, food insecurity).
- Biochemical data, Medical Tests, and Procedures: Laboratory data (A1c, lipid profile, kidney function).
- Anthropometric Measurements: Height, weight, body mass index (BMI), growth rate, and rate of weight change.
- Nutrition-focused physical finders: General physical appearance, body language, digestive system, and blood pressure.

Nutrition Intervention:

- Implement MNT selecting from a variety of nutrition interventions to help patients achieve individualized nutrition goals.
- Encourage consumption of macronutrients based on Dietary Reference Intakes for healthy children and adults.
- Implement nutrition education and counseling with emphasis on the recommendations from the major and contributing factors to nutrition therapy.

Nutrition Monitoring and Evaluation:

- Coordinate care with an interdisciplinary team.
- Monitor and evaulate food intake, medication, metabolic control, anthropometric measurements and physical activity.
- Use blood glucose monitoring results to evaluate the achievement of goals and effectiveness of MNT. Glucose monitoring results can help determine whether food and/or medication need to be adjusted.

STRATEGIES FOR TYPE 1 DIABETES

The following strategies are the starting points for the nutrition component of intensified management for people with type 1 diabetes. They form the basis of care, regardless of the specific meal-planning approach used.

- Insulin therapy should be integrated into an indivdual's dietary and physical activity pattern.
- Individuals using rapid-acting insulin either by injection or an insulin pump should adjust the meal and snack insulin doses based on the carbohydrate of their meals and snacks.
- For individuals using fixed daily insulin doses, daily carbohydrate intake should be kept consistent with respect to time and amount.
- For planned exercise, insulin doses can be adjusted. For unplanned exercise, extra carbohydrate may be needed.

Maintaining a consistent carbohydrate intake for individuals on fixed daily insulin doses can be extremely challenging. On presentation, newly diagnosed individuals with type 1 diabetes have often experienced weight loss and and an increase in appetite with the initiation of insulin therapy. Therefore, it is important to base the initial diabetes meal plan on the patient's appetite in order to restore and/or maintain appropriate body weight and allow for normal growth and development. Once the initial meal plan has been established, it is important to monitor weight, blood pressure, A1c, lipids, and other clinical parameters to determine if further modifications are needed to meet goals.

For individuals using either multiple daily injections (MDI) or continuous subcutaneous insulin infusion (CSII), lifestyle flexibility and maintaining optimal blood glucose control is achieved by developing personal algorithms that take into account the interplay of insulin, food intake and exercise. Using these algorithms, patients are able to systematically adjust therapy as needed in response to deviations from usual patterns.

Two different approaches can be used when a patient initiates this type of intensive diabetes management. One approach involves prescribing a consistent carbohydrate meal plan based primarily on the patient's usual intake. The patient should follow the prescribed meal plan until the insulin dosages are adjusted to achieve target glycemia levels. After the optimal insulin dosage for each meal is established, the insulin dose per quantity of carbohydrate (insulin-to-carbohydrate ratio) can be determined. For example: If a patient consistently eats a lunch containing about 72g of carbohydrate and requires 8 units of rapid-acting insulin when the pre-lunch blood glucose level is at target, this patient requires 1 unit of insulin for every 9g of carbohydrate at lunch (72 divided by 8). This formula, expressed as a ratio, can then be used to determine insulin needed for different amounts of carbohydrate at lunchtime. Ratios for breakfast, dinner, and snacks can be calculated in the same way. It is normal for patients to have different insulin-to-carbohydrate ratios for different meals.

For patients skilled in carbohydrate counting but who have difficulty eating consistent amounts of carbohydrate, a second approach uses a formula to determine the insulin to carbohydrate ratio. This approach is known as the 500 rule:

divide 500 by the total daily insulin dose. For example, a patient whose total daily insulin dose is 50 units would divide 500 by 50 to achieve a ratio of 1:10. This ratio may then need to be adjusted ("fine tuned") based on evaluation of postprandial blood glucose levels and food records.

These strategies arise from a strong scientific and behavioral base and describe a much less prescriptive approach than has been commonly used in the past. They acknowledge the difficulty in changing ingrained food habits, the wide range of diets that can be compatible with good diabetes control, and the importance of prioritizing the patient's preferences and lifestyle values while supporting increased flexibility and patient choice to the overall plan of care. Like other aspects of intensified management, they require more time and skill on the part of health care providers and patients than do more traditional approaches.

STRATEGIES FOR TYPE 2 DIABETES

For patients with type 2 diabetes, the primary focus of MNT is on weight loss and lifestyle strategies to improve abnormalities in glucose, lipid, and blood pressure and to reduce the risk of chronic complications, especially cardiovascular disease. Near-normal blood glucose control reduces insulin resistance and preserves insulin secretory capacity in type 2 diabetes. Hypocaloric diets and modest weight loss (5–7% of body weight) often improve glycemic control in the short-term and, if maintained, can contribute to long-term improvements in glycemic contol. Modest weight loss has been shown to improve insulin resistance in overweight (body mass index [BMI] ≥ 25 kg/m^2) and obese (BMI ≥ 30 kg/m^2) insulin resistant individuals. The risk of comorbidity increases with BMIs in this range and higher. Waist circumference is used as a measure of visceral fat. A waist circumference of ≥35 inches in women and ≥40 inches in men is used in conjunction with BMI to assess the risk of cardiovascular disease as well as the risk for type 2 diabetes.

Unfortunately, generally effective strategies for long-term maintenance of weight loss are unknown, and long-term weight loss is difficult for most people to achieve. Low carbohydrate or low fat calorie-restricted diets may be effective for weight loss in the short term (up to 1 year). Physical activity and behavior modification are important components of weight loss programs and are adjuncts to MNT in maintaining weight loss.

A structured, intensive lifestyle program that encompasses education, counseling, behavioral therapy, reduced calorie and fat intake (<30% of total calories), regular and sustained physical activity, and frequent contact with health care providers are requirements to achieve a 5–7% weight loss. Physical activity alone has only a modest effect on weight loss, but is nevertheless important for improving insulin sensitivity, lowering blood glucose levels, and maintaining long-term weight loss. A weight loss plan of 500–1,000 fewer calories per week will initially result in a loss of approximately 1–2 pounds per week. However, without continued support and follow-up, the weight is often regained.

Traditionally, low-fat diets have been prescribed for overweight or obese people with type 2 diabetes. Because weight loss is difficult to sustain, other approaches have recently been explored, including low-carbohydrate diets. There is evidence that very low-carbohydrate diets may, in the short term, result in more weight loss than low-fat diets. However, in the longer term, differences in weight loss between very low-carbohydrate and low-fat diets are not significant, and weight loss is modest with both dietary approaches. The long-term effects of very low-carbohydrate diets are unknown; these diets may be deficient in fiber, vitamins, and minerals and usually rate low on palatability, thus making it difficult to sustain for a long period of time. A moderate reduction in carbohydrate can be considered for people with type 2 diabetes and may be more efficacious.

Meal replacements are another dietary approach that may be considered for the overweight or obese patient with type 2 diabetes. Meal replacements, typically consisting of shakes or prepackaged meals, can be safely used for one or two meals per day. They provide a defined amount of calories and nutrients and can result in significant weight loss. Use of meal replacements generally must be continued, however, to sustain the weight loss.

Conversely, very low calorie diets (VLCDs) that provide ≤800 calories per day are not typically recommended as a weight loss approach, despite the fact that they do result in significant weight loss and improved glycemic and lipid control. Long-term use of VLCD use can be detrimental to good health and, when VLCDs are stopped, weight is quickly regained. If a VLCD is considered, it must be part of a structured program that provides ongoing support.

Weight loss medications have been used in combination with lifestyle changes to successfully promote weight loss (5–10%) among overweight or obese individuals with type 2 diabetes. Pharmacological therapy should only be used in patients with a BMI > 27 kg/m². For individuals with a BMI ≥ 35 kg/m², bariatric surgery has been shown to be an effective weight loss treatment that can result in marked improvement in glycemia and cardiovascular risk factors, with the exception of hypercholesterolemia. The risks of bariatric surgery are serious and may include increased mortality, blood clots, hernia, infection, and dumping syndrome.

The following strategies form the basis for dietary intervention in all people with type 2 diabetes. When applied in conjunction with active monitoring of glucose, they also delineate the nutrition component of intensified management for this group.

- The nutrition prescription should be based on the lifestyle changes that patients are willing and able to make.
- Review the patient's usual intake with respect to total energy, food and carbohydrate distribution throughout the day, fat intake (type and amounts), and food selection.
- Distribute food throughout the day to eliminate large concentrations of calories or carbohydrate that may contribute to postprandial glucose elevation.
- Make recommendations regarding improvement in food choices to comprise a nutritionally adequate meal plan with reduced total, saturated, and trans fat, if needed.
- Advise patients regarding cholesterol intake per guidelines (Table 9.3).
- If the patient is overweight, recommend moderate calorie restriction (no more than 250–500 kcal/day below current intake) and regular physical

Table 9.5 Using Blood Glucose Monitoring to Fine-Tune Nutrition Therapy

Type of Diabetes	Pharmacological Management	Blood Glucose Monitoring Schedule	Question to Ask	Strategy to Correct Elevated Blood Glucose
Type 2, obese	None; oral diabetes medication(s), incretin mimetic, or insulin	Fasting	Does the overnight insulin or other oral glucose-lowering agent suppress hepatic glucose output sufficiently to produce desired fasting blood glucose level?	Reduce total calories; review bedtime snack and any other foods eaten overnight. Evaluate pharmacological management.
		2–3-hour postprandial or next pre-meal blood glucose	Does available insulin (endogenous or exogenous) cover the meal eaten, producing the desire postprandial value?	Reduce calories and/or carbohydrate/fat in meal. When obesity is present, food reduction and/or increased physical activity are preferred to increases in medication whenever possible. Consider the glycemic impacrt of carbohydrate ingested.
Type 1 or Type 2, non-obese	Insulin	Fasting	Does overnight exogenous insulin suppress hepatic glucose output sufficiently to produce desired fasting blood glucose level?	Adjust dose or timing of overnight insulin; review bedtime snack and any other foods eaten overnight. Consider adding another oral glucose-lowering agent or an incretin mimetic in type 2 patients. Insulin coverage may be needed for bedtime snack in those patients on CSII or MDI therapy.
		2–3-hours postprandial (rapid-acting insulin analog) or next pre-meal value (regular insulin)	Is the pre-meal insulin dose appropriate?	Adjust dose or timing of pre-meal insulin; fine-tune patient's insulin algorithm; evaluate method used to quantify carbohydrate and glycemic impact (GI/GL) of carbohydrate eaten.
		Pre-meal (CSII or MDI only)	Is the basal insulin dose or rate (CSII) correct?	Adjust basal insulin to bring pre-meal blood glucose into target range.

Table 9.6 Adjusting Meal Bolus Dose Based on Rate of Glucose Change

- If glucose is decreasing 1–2 mg/dl/min, subtract 10% from calculated meal bolus
- If glucose is decreasing >2 mg/dl/min, subtract 20% from calculated meal bolus
- If glucose is increasing 1–2 mg/dl/min, add 10% to calculated meal bolus
- If glucose is increasing >2 mg/dl/min, add 20% to calculated meal bolus

activity to help promote modest, gradual weight loss. Calorie restriction is a valuable glucose control strategy for many people with type 2 diabetes, whether or not weight loss is achieved.

- Monitor blood glucose and adjust food distribution, portions, and selection (as needed) in concert with medications and exercise, to achieve glucose goals.
- Monitor weight, blood pressure, A1c, lipids, and other clinical parameters and modify the initial meal plan as needed to meet goals.

Traditionally defined "desirable" or "ideal" body weight is no longer used in setting weight goals for diabetes patients. The guideline terminology "reasonable weight" refers to the weight an individual and his or her health care provider agree can be achieved and maintained, in both the short and long term. In addition, goals for BMI and waist circumference, mutually agreed upon by the patient and practitioner, may be more achievable and realistic than focusing on a predetermined body weight goal.

In overweight people with type 2 diabetes, modest weight loss on the order of 10–15 lb (5–7 kg), regardless of starting weight, is often associated with significant improvements in glycemic, lipid, and blood pressure control. Improved glycemia is more likely to occur relatively early in the course of the disease while patients retain the capacity to produce effective levels of endogenous insulin. Patients who do not experience an improvement in glucose control with a weight loss in this range are unlikely to see any beneficial effect on glucose control with additional weight loss alone. Persistent fasting hyperglycemia despite a 10-lb (5-kg) weight loss suggests the need for initiation of, or changes in, pharmacological therapy. In addition, because glucose control is the primary goal of therapy, an oral glucose-lowering agent (sulfonylurea, biguanide, or meglitinide, thiazolidimedione, alpha glucosidase or dipetidyl peptidase–4 in [DPP–4] inhibitor). Incretin mimetic therapy (exenatide or liraglutide) or insulin should be considered when glucose control has not improved despite better nutrition and exercise, whether or not weight loss has occurred.

GLUCOSE MONITORING AND THE NUTRITION PLAN

BLOOD GLUCOSE MONITORING

Appropriate use of the results of blood glucose monitoring plays an essential role in the nutrition aspects of intensive diabetes management. Blood glucose monitoring provides the feedback needed to fine-tune the meal plan in concert with physical activity, medications (if used), and other relevant factors.

When evaluated in relation to food records, blood glucose monitoring can be used to refine the dietary approach in various ways. Postprandial glucose values can guide modification of the basic meal plan or can be used to tailor the patient's insulin-to-carbohydrate ratio or insulin adjustment algorithm. Review of food records in conjunction with glucose results reveals the effect of various single foods and food combinations. Such information, when used as the basis for determining prandial insulin dosing, can increase the patient's flexibility in food choices while maintaining or improving glucose control. Some sample monitoring strategies that help to fine-tune nutritional care are outlined in Table 9.5.

In overweight or obese patients with type 2 diabetes, the primary strategy to restore postprandial glucose values to the target range is to decrease calories and/or carbohydrate. Conversely, in people with type 1 diabetes and in patients of normal weight who have type 2 diabetes and are treated with insulin, the primary strategy for preventing or correcting postprandial glucose elevations is to modify the dose and/or timing of the meal-related insulin dose to match the food consumed. However, a decrease in carbohydrate intake at the meal should also be considered. Figure 9.1 illustrates schematically the process of nutrition intervention in intensive management, including the essential role of blood glucose monitoring in evaluating and adjusting intervention.

CONTINUOUS GLUCOSE MONITORING (CGM)

Real-time continuous glucose monitoring (RT-CGM) systems a subcutaneous glucose sensor to measure interstitial glucose concentrations. They provide detailed information on glucose patterns and trends, including postprandial glucose values that are difficult to ascertain by episodic monitoring of blood glucose concentrations. They also provide information on the direction of rate and change of glucose concentrations. By allowing patients to observe glucose values and trends as they occur, RT-CGM provides the patient with the opportunity to make immediate decisions based on real-time glucose values and perform more immediate therapy adjustments. For example, meal boluses can be

---

Table 9.7 Nutrition Factors Contributing to Hypoglycemia

- Omitting or delaying planned meals or snacks
- Inappropriate timing of insulin relative to meals
- Imbalance between food and meal-related insulin dose because of:
  - inaccurate estimation of carbohydrate intake when calculating meal-related boluses
  - consuming less carbohydrate than usual without adjusting insulin dose
- Inadequate carbohydrate supplementation or medication adjustment for physical activity
- Consuming alcohol without food
- Delayed absorption of carbohydrate when eating high-fat or low-glycemic-index meals and using a rapid-acting insulin analog

adjusted based on the premeal rate of glucose change. A sample algorithm for this purpose is shown in Table 9.6.

The data obtained from RT-CGM also allow for greater precision in matching the dose and timing of mealtime insulin to postprandial glucose profiles. RT-CGM can be especially helpful for adjusting the insulin dose for meals that produce complex postmeal glucose profiles (e.g., pizza). RT-CGM can be used to identify a problematic postmeal glucose pattern and then to monitor the postprandial pattern following various corrective bolusing schemes. In this way, the optimal dose and time parameters for the meal insulin bolus can be determined.

RT-CGM data can be an important tool for reshaping eating behavior as patients receive immediate feedback on their personal glycemic responses to their food choices. RT-CGM has made it possible for users to more clearly see that the food factors that determine the postprandial glucose profile include not only the amount of carbohydrate but also the type of carbohydrate (i.e., glycemic index value), and the effect of fat, caffeine, and alcohol. Foods with a high glycemic index may cause a postprandial glucose spike because of a mismatch between the rapid absorption of the carbohydrate and the less rapid onset of action of the insulin bolus. Fat can affect postprandial glucose levels by slowing gastric emptying, thereby delaying the increase in postmeal glucose levels, and also by decreasing postprandial insulin sensitivity, leading to higher postmeal glucose levels than would be produced by a carbohydrate-equivalent low-fat meal. Caffeine, like fat, can reduce insulin sensitivity in some people, also leading to higher glucose levels. Alcohol has a glucose-lowering effect, as it blocks glucose release from the liver. However, alcoholic beverages containing significant carbohydrate may initially cause an increase followed by a later decrease in glucose levels. The multiplicity of food factors affecting postprandial glucose levels can make diabetes control challenging for the patient. However, by providing feedback on glycemic responses to various food factors, RT-CGM can enable the motivated patient to improve improved glycemic control with less frequent hypoglycemia.

All RT-CGM systems currently approved for patient use require calibration using a conventional blood glucose meter, and interstitial glucose values require confirmation using a blood glucose meter before treatment decisions are enacted.

HYPOGLYCEMIA

Nutrition strategies are important for the prevention of hypoglycemia in all people whose diabetes treatment includes insulin or an insulin secretagogue. Common nutrition factors that contribute to hypoglycemia risk are listed in Table 9.7, and issues and strategies relative to each factor are discussed next.

OMITTING OR DELAYING PLANNED MEALS OR SNACKS

The risk of hypoglycemia from omitting or delaying meals is greatest in patients who use insulin regimens that include intermediate- and short-acting (regular) insulin. The increased risk is attributable to high circulating insulin levels between meals and overnight owing to the time–action profiles of intermediate- and short-acting insulin. The risk of hypoglycemia is also high if meals or snacks are omitted or delayed in patients using MDI regimens or in patients using an insulin secreta-gogue. Patients whose diabetes is treated by diet alone or those who use oral glucose-lowering agents such as biguanides,pioglitazone, or dipetidyl peptidase–4 inhibitors [DPP–4] as monotherapy are not at increased risk of hypoglycemia when meals are delayed or omitted.

The risk for hypoglycemia should be considered when selecting a pharmaco-logical regimen. Individuals whose work or other activities make it difficult to predict or control meal times (e.g., trial lawyers, inpatient medical staff, traveling salespeople) will have less frequent hypoglycemia using insulin regimens that allow more meal time flexibility.

All patients whose diabetes treatment includes insulin or an insulin secreta-gogue should receive education regarding appropriate meal timing for their par-ticular regimen. Carrying a source of rapidly absorbed carbohydrate is a vital self-management behavior for all such patients to prevent hypoglycemia, particu-larly when meals are unavoidably delayed.

INAPPROPRIATE TIMING OF INSULIN RELATIVE TO MEALS

The risk for hypoglycemia is greatest when the peak action of insulin is not synchronized with the peak of glucose entry into the bloodstream after a meal. A common scenario: the patient takes a bolus of short-acting insulin immediately before eating. Hyperglycemia occurs in the immediate postprandial period, because carbohydrate is absorbed but insulin has not yet reached its peak action. Two to three hours later, when little or no carbohydrate is entering the circulation and insulin action has reached its peak, blood glucose levels decrease and hypogly-cemia may occur. Delaying the meal results in a better match between insulin action and postprandial glucose availability but is difficult for many patients to implement. Rapid-acting insulin analogs (lispro, aspart, glulisine), which achieve their peak action earlier than regular insulin, shorten the interval between admin-istering the bolus and eating the meal. The shorter total duration of action of these insulins also reduces the risk for between-meal and nocturnal hypoglycemia. When intermediate-acting insulin is injected in the morning, it is necessary to schedule lunch at the time when this insulin is peaking to reduce the risk of pre-lunch hypoglycemia. Blood glucose monitoring should be used to confirm optional insulin timing relative to meals because the action profiles of specific insulin preparations vary considerably from person to person, and are further affected by injection site, exercise, and other factors.

In addition to modifying insulin administration or meal timing, another strategy for minimizing risk for hypoglycemia between meals is to include snacks in the meal plan. Snacks are often needed to prevent hypoglycemia in individuals using split mixed regimens (see Multi-Component Insulin Regimens) because of the broad peak action curves of short-acting and intermediate-acting insulin (Neutral Prot-amine Hagedorn, NPH). The need for snacks often can be eliminated by using rapid-acting insulin analogs in combination with a long-acting insulin, either glargine or detemir, to provide between-meal insulin coverage.

IMBALANCE BETWEEN FOOD AND MEAL-RELATED INSULIN DOSE

Hypoglycemia may result when the meal-related insulin dose is too large relative to the amount of food eaten. In the intensively managed MDI or CSII patient who adjusts premeal boluses for anticipated intake, hypoglycemia most often occurs because of errors in estimating food and/or carbohydrate intake. Bolus calculations can be based on carbohydrate choices, carbohydrate intake, or known meal composition (menus), but irrespective of the method used, the algorithm used must be individualized to the patient. Most people benefit from a period of weighing and measuring their food to train their eye to accurately estimate portion sizes.

Unless the blood glucose level is decreasing rapidly, the meal insulin bolus should be given before starting the meal. However, in special circumstances, it may be advisable to inject the meal bolus at the end of a meal. Doing so allows more calibration of the bolus to the actual amount eaten and is particularly helpful in the management of young children with diabetes and during illness or pregnancy, when nausea may interfere with eating.

For patients on a fixed insulin plan, it must be remembered that a fixed meal plan is required. If one parameter changes, the other must reflect this change. Although not all patients will choose to increase insulin doses to accommodate extra food intake—perhaps as a means of weight management—they should at least be given instruction on how to prevent hypoglycemia if a smaller-than-normal meal is eaten. Individualized guidelines for insulin reduction could be used, or the missing carbohydrate could be replaced with another equivalent carbohydrate source, such as fruit or a snack.

INADEQUATE FOOD SUPPLEMENTATION FOR EXERCISE

Blood glucose monitoring is required to calibrate insulin doses and/or carbohydrate intake to reduce hypoglycemia risk with exercise. The decision whether to adjust food or insulin is determined by the individual's diabetes management goals and is affected by whether the exercise is planned. When exercise is planned, it is preferable to reduce the dose of insulin acting during the period of physical activity to minimize hypoglycemia risk (see Chapter 6, Multiple-Component Insulin Regimens).

If exercise is not planned with sufficient time to permit insulin dose adjustment, additional carbohydrate is usually needed to prevent exercise-related hypoglycemia. Depending on the blood glucose level at the start of exercise, as well as the intensity and duration of the activity, the extra carbohydrate may be taken before, during, and/or after exercise. If blood glucose levels are less than 100 mg/dl before starting exercise, carbohydrate should be ingested before the activity begins. During exercise of moderate intensity, glucose uptake is increased by 2–3 mg/kg/min or about 8–13 g/h, which supports the general recommendation to add 15 g carbohydrate for every 30–60 minutes of activity exceeding the patient's usual level of physical activity. Patients will need personalized guidelines based on blood glucose monitoring to guide carbohydrate supplementation for exercise. When exercise has been intense or prolonged, the risk for hypoglycemia extends

Table 9.8 Sample Personal Algorithm for Treatment of Hypoglycemia

Each 5 g of glucose increases your blood glucose ~15 mg/dl. Your goal blood glucose after treatment of hypoglycemia is about 120 mg/dl.

If your blood glucose is:	Eat this much glucose:
<40	30 g
40–50	25 g
51–60	20 g
61–70	15 g
>70 with symptoms	5–10 g

for up to 24 hours postexercise. Therefore, additional snacks may be needed in the hours after exercise and before bedtime, when strenuous exercise has occurred in the afternoon or evening. Reduction of the amount of insulin administered after particularly lengthy or intense exercise is also required.

Exercise is a central component of the overall management of individuals attempting to reach and maintain a reasonable body weight. It is obviously preferable to avoid increasing food intake to cover exercise in such individuals. To better support weight management and calorie restriction goals, exercise can be scheduled after meals when blood glucose levels are peaking. If exercising after meals is not possible, or if it does not prevent hypoglycemia, medication doses should be decreased to allow exercise to occur without having to increase food intake.

CONSUMING ALCOHOL ON AN EMPTY STOMACH

Alcohol inhibits gluconeogenesis and interferes with the counterregulatory response to insulin-induced hypoglycemia. Therefore, alcohol may contribute to hypoglycemia, especially in people with type 1 diabetes. If sweet wines, liqueurs, or drinks made with regular soda or fruit juices are consumed, the carbohydrate may need to be included in the calculation of the meal bolus. This calculation should be done cautiously though because of the hypoglycemia risk associated with alcohol. Choosing dry wines, light beers, and drinks made with noncaloric mixers may simplify the management of alcohol consumption in people with diabetes who choose to consume alcohol. Checking the blood glucose level before going to sleep is a recommended safety precaution for patients who have been drinking alcohol.

Because they typically are insulin resistant, alcohol-induced hypoglycemia is less of a risk in people with type 2 diabetes, unless they are using insulin or an insulin secretagogue to manage their diabetes.

Table 9.9 Benefits and Drawbacks of Major Types of Meal-Planning Systems

System type	Description	Benefits	Drawbacks
General guidelines	USDA Choose My Plate Guidelines; Dietary Guidelines for Americans	Easy to understand Good initial teaching tools Focus on healthy food choices	Low emphasis on measuring portions complicates coordinating insulin doses with food
Menu planning	Written out sample menus	Specific Simple to use Can guide food choices while patient learns more advanced concepts Can use patient's preferred and available foods	Lack of flexibility to respond to unusual circumstances Keeps decision making in hands of caregiver instead of patient
Exchange/choice	Lists that group foods of similar nutritional content, indicating portions of each that can be substituted to provide variety; accompanied by a meal pattern that indicates the number of servings to be eaten from each group at each meal	Includes portion control Facilitates calorie adjustment Supports widely available materials such as food lists, recipes, and menus Multiple nutrition concerns can be incorporated into a single plan	Exchange concept is difficult for many to understand Time-consuming to teach Can be limiting and prescriptive, especially if inadequate education is provided Does not always correlate with portions listed on food labels
Counting	Systems that focus on counting amounts of given nutrients: common ones are carbohydrate counting for glucose control and fat counting for calorie control/weight management	Allows greatest flexibility in food choices Emphasis is on carefully quantifying food intake Simple to teach and apply because of single-topic focus Carbohydrate counting is the most common method for matching insulin to food intake	Other nutrition concepts (i.e., healthy food choices or cardiovascular risk reduction) must be taught separately Difficult for patients who are cognitively impaired or learning disabled

ORAL TREATMENT OF HYPOGLYCEMIA

Helping each patient develop a personally calibrated treatment plan for hypoglycemia is a valuable strategy to promote better blood glucose control. Overtreatment of hypoglycemia is common and is often caused by a lack of or inadequate advice on appropriate treatment of hypoglycemia. When the same "take 15–20 g of carbohydrate" advice is given to all patients, the result will be inadequate treatment in some circumstances and excessive treatment in others. The increase in blood glucose level produced by a given amount of carbohydrate varies from person to person, primarily as a result of differences in body size and insulin sensitivity. For example, a given quantity of carbohydrate will generally increase the blood glucose level more in a small person than it will in a larger person.

To develop an individualized hypoglycemia treatment algorithm for a patient, begin with the estimate that each 5 g of glucose increases blood glucose ~20 mg/dl (1.1 mmol/l; an approximate value for a 150-lb [69-kg] person). With subsequent blood glucose monitoring, fine-tune this value, based on the patient's response to given amounts of glucose. For example, suppose a 100-lb (45-kg) woman finds that her blood glucose level is 40 mg/dl (2.2 mmol/l), and she wants to increase her blood glucose level by ~60 mg/dl (3.3 mmol/l) to 100 mg/dl (5.6 mmol/l). If she treats the hypoglycemia with 15 g carbohydrate expecting that each 5 g carbohydrate will increase her blood glucose 20 mg/dl but instead her blood glucose increases to 145 mg/dl (8.0 mmol/l), this demonstrates that every 5 g of glucose increases her blood glucose by 35 mg/dl. When the effect of a specific amount of ingested glucose is known, an algorithm can be developed, as illustrated in Table 9.8. The patient can then calibrate treatment of any subsequent episode of hypoglycemia based on the current blood glucose concentration and a personal blood glucose target. Providing the patient with an algorithm can avoid a potential source of treatment error because it eliminates the patient's need to perform calculations in a hypoglycemic state.

Virtually any nonfat source of carbohydrate (e.g., saltines, regular soda, fruit juice, nonfat milk) can be used to treat hypoglycemia; however, glucose is the most rapid-acting carbohydrate source. Commercially prepared products, such as glucose tablets and glucose gels, are higher in available glucose than are most high-carbohydrate foods, and they offer the additional advantages of more precise glucose dosing and a more predictable blood glucose response than food sources of carbohydrate.

FACILITATING NUTRITION SELF-MANAGEMENT

Achieving optimal glycemic control requires that the patient successfully balance food intake, insulin, and physical activity. Rigid or strict diets are generally not conducive to achieving glycemic control, as they are not individualized to the unique characteristics, preferences, and lifestyle of the patient. In addition, most people are unable to sustain a structured eating plan for any significant length of time. Each patient who uses an intensified management approach must receive the depth of education required to build nutrition self-management skills.

As previously described, this process begins with a nutrition assessment to enable the dietitian to tailor MNT to each patient's unique circumstances. The ensuing educational process progresses from the mutual identification of specific goals through appropriate stepwise intervention and is guided throughout by evaluation of the patient's knowledge and skill, as well as by clinical parameters. These processes of assessment and education are similar for every patient, regardless of the specific approach to diabetes meal planning used.

MEAL-PLANNING APPROACHES FOR INTENSIFIED MANAGEMENT

Several distinct meal-planning systems are commonly used in diabetes MNT. Each stresses a different factor (e.g., calories, portion control, food choices, fat or carbohydrate content). The DCCT demonstrated that many different approaches to meal planning can be used successfully in intensive management regimens. The four major types of diabetes meal-planning systems and the benefits of each are summarized in Table 9.9. The choice of a specific meal-planning approach should be based on a review of the patient's current intake and food choices, clinical goals, learning style, and desire for flexibility.

It is important to consider the amount of time necessary to teach various meal-planning approaches. Sufficient and effective patient education and support materials must be available. Similarly, all approaches entail a staged program of education, progressing from simple concepts of diabetes nutrition management to the more in-depth knowledge that supports nutrition self-management and informed decision making.

CARBOHYDRATE COUNTING

Carbohydrate counting is a meal planning system that involves determining the amount (measured in grams) of carbohydrate eaten at a meal or a snack. Because dietary carbohydrate is the chief determinant of meal-related insulin requirement, it is important to be able to correctly identify the amount of carbohydrate in food for accurate insulin dosing. Patients can learn to count specific grams of carbohydrate or carbohydrate choices, where one choice is equivalent to 15 g carbohydrate. Carbohydrate counting can be used as the sole meal-planning approach or in concert with other systems to fine-tune blood glucose control. The

Table 9.10 Prevention of Weight Gain During Intensive Management

- Reduce calore intake by 250–500 kcal/d
- Eliminate between-meal snacks
- Treat hypoglycemia with measured amounts of glucose
- Initiate or increase physical activity
- Decrease insulin for exercise instead of snacking
- Educate on flexibility in meal planning

health care provider can also use carbohydrate counting to determine the cause of unexplained blood glucose control problems.

For patients on MDI regimens or CSII, use of advanced carbohydrate counting skills are encouraged. This method attempts to more precisely count carbohydrates in foods and match insulin doses based on anticipated or consumed carbohydrate intake. To determine the ratio of insulin needed for the amount of carbohydrate consumed, initially, basic carbohydrate counting can be implemented as a stable meal plan with a given quantity of carbohydrate for each meal and snack, preferably based on the patient's typical intake. During this initial period on a meal plan, the patient weighs and measures food portions (to gain skill in visually estimating portion sizes), reads food labels, and maintains complete food and blood glucose records. Evaluation of this data allows for the patient's insulin-to-carbohydrate ratio to be determined (i.e., the ratio between the grams of carbohydrate eaten and the number of units of mealtime insulin required). The insulin-to-carbohydrate ratio for adults with type 1 diabetes is commonly in the range 1:10–1:15 (1 unit of insulin for each 10–15 g carbohydrate); however, this generalization cannot be made for every patient to optimize blood glucose control. The precise ratio for each patient is determined by reviewing food records and blood glucose monitoring results. For additional information on carbohydrate counting, refer to Practical Carbohydrate Counting: A How-to-Teach Guide for Health Professionals (see Bibliography).

Although uncommon, some patients achieve better blood glucose control when they also account for the effect of dietary protein and fat on their blood glucose levels; however, this approach should be used with caution in people using rapid-acting insulin. Any glucose derived from dietary protein appears in the bloodstream in the late postprandial period and by including protein in bolus calculations for rapid-acting insulin analogs, one may increase the risk for hypoglycemia in the immediate postprandial period. One strategy to offset this risk is to deliver the insulin bolus after the meal is eaten. For patients using insulin pumps, advanced bolus options ("dual," "combo," "extended," and "square-wave" boluses) enable patients to deliver a portion of the insulin bolus after the meal to better match the effect of protein on blood glucose levels.

Furthermore, some patients are able to establish an insulin-to-fat ratio based on experience and careful observation of the effects of fat on postprandial glucose levels. RT-CGM can be a valuable tool in such advanced meal-planning techniques. The insulin-to-fat ratio can be used to augment the bolus dose calculated on the basis of the carbohydrate content (and, in some cases, the protein content) of the meal. The effects of dietary fat (delayed digestion of carbohydrate and decreased postprandial insulin sensitivity), similar to those of protein, occur in the late postprandial period. Therefore, to offset the effect of fat, bolus insulin must be delivered after the meal to avoid postprandial hypoglycemia and is best achieved using the advanced bolus options of an insulin pump.

WEIGHT GAIN ASSOCIATED WITH INTENSIVE MANAGEMENT

Weight gain may accompany intensive management when optimal blood glucose control is achieved, and it affects patients regardless of age or sex. Factors thought to be associated with weight gain are failure to compensate for calories no longer lost via glycosuria, consumption of extra calories to treat more frequent episodes of hypoglycemia, and/or repletion of body water or protein lost during a period of poor glucose control. In addition, patients on intensive therapy may find that they can consume a greater variety of foods without loss of glucose control and, therefore, experience the same result from overeating as the rest of the population.

PREVENTION

Experience suggests that the following strategies may be helpful (Table 9.10):

■ **Reduce caloric intake at the initiation of intensive management.** A detailed nutrition history should be used to negotiate a meal plan that is 250–500 kcal less than that consumed before intensification of therapy, depending on degree of control before undertaking intensive management. The rationale for this change should be carefully explained.

■ **Eliminate between-meal snacks.** For many patients, traditional between-meal snacks necessitated by use of insulin regimens based on the use of intermediate-acting and/or regular insulin are one of the inconveniences of diabetes management. Many patients are willing to eliminate snacks as a means of reducing caloric intake. A consistent need for snacks between meals to avoid hypoglycemia may indicate that the basal insulin dose is excessive. Children and adolescents may need snacks to provide appropriate calories for normal growth. Most young children have a snack in the middle of the morning, in the afternoon, and may eat again before going to bed. Older children and adolescents generally have an after-school snack and may or may not have a snack before bed.

■ **Treat hypoglycemia with glucose.** Treating hypoglycemia with foods that contain fat and/or protein in addition to carbohydrate slows the correction of hypoglycemia and leads to increased caloric intake. Therefore, patients should be urged to avoid treating hypoglycemia with common snack foods such as cheese and crackers or candy bars. The appropriate amount of carbohydrate (measured in grams) should be consumed to correct the hypoglycemia.

■ **Initiate an exercise program as part of intensive management.** The type and amount of exercise should be individualized. Current exercise recommendations for most adults are to aim for at least 30 minutes of moderate-intensity activity on most, if not all, days of the week, or approximately 150 minutes of exercise per week. The exercise program should also include resistance exercise, in addition to aerobic exercise, which can improve insulin sensitivity in people with type 2 diabetes.

■ **Decrease insulin doses for activity that exceeds daily routines.** Traditional dogma has taught patients to eat more when they exercise more than usual, a practice that makes weight control more difficult. With practice and judicious use of blood glucose monitoring, patients can become skilled at reducing the usual insulin dose to offset the effect of additional exercise.

■ **Educate o flexibility in meal planning.** Patients can be educated on strategies to reduce their food intake for convenience or weight control and to appropriately adjust insulin doses.

BIBLIOGRAPHY

American Diabetes Association: Nutrition recommendations and interventions for diabetes. A position statement of the American Diabetes Association. *Diabetes Care* 31 (Suppl. 1):S61–S78, 2008

American Diabetes Association/American Dietetic Association: *Advanced Carbohydrate Counting*. Alexandria, VA, American Diabetes Association, and Chicago, American Dietetic Association, 2010

American Diabetes Association/American Dietetic Association: *Basic Carbohydrate Counting*. Alexandria, VA, American Diabetes Association, and Chicago, American Dietetic Association, 2010

Delahanty LM, Halford BN: The role of diet behaviors in achieving improved glycemic control in intensively treated patients in the Diabetes Control and Complications Trial. *Diabetes Care* 16:1453–1458, 1993

Diabetes Control and Complications Trial (DCCT) Research Group: Weight gain associated with intensive therapy in the Diabetes Control and Complications Trial. *Diabetes Care* 11:567–573, 1988

Diabetes Control and Complications Trial (DCCT) Research Group: Nutrition interventions for intensive therapy in the Diabetes Control and Complications Trial. *J Am Diet Assoc* 93:768–772, 1993

Diabetes Control and Complications Trial (DCCT) Research Group: Expanded role of the dietitian in the Diabetes Control and Complications Trial: implications for clinical practice. *J Am Diet Assoc* 93:758–767, 1994

Franz MJ, Boucher JL, Green-Pastors J, Power MA: Evidence-based nutrition practice guidelines for diabetes and scope and standards of practice. *J Am Diet Assoc* 108 (Suppl.): S52–S58, 2008

Garg S, Zisser H, Schwartz S, Bailey T, Kaplan R, Ellis S, Jovanovic L: Improvement in glycemic excursions with a transcutaneous, real-time continuous glucose sensor: a randomized control trial. *Diabetes Care* 29:44–50, 2006

Juvenile Diabetes Research Foundation Continuous Glucose Monitoring Study Group; Tamborlane WV, Beck RW, Bode BW, Buckingham B, Chase HP, Clemons R, Fiallo-Scharer R, Fox LA, Gilliam LK, Hirsch IB, Huang ES, Kollman C, Kowalski AJ, Laffel L, Lawrence JM, Lee J, Mauras N, O'Grady M, Ruedy KJ, Tansey M, Tsalikian E, Weinzimer S, Wilson DM, Wolpert H, Wysocki T, Xing D: Continuous glucose monitoring and intensive treatment of type 1 diabetes. *N Engl J Med* 359(14):1464–76, 2008

Look AHEAD Research Group; PI-Sunyer X, Blackburn G, Brancati FL, et. al.: Long-term effects of a lifestyle intervention on weight and cardiovascular risk factors in individuals with type 2 diabetes mellitus: Four-year results of the Look AHEAD trial. *Arch Intern Med* 170(17): 1566–1575, 2010

Warshaw H, Bolderman K: *Practical Carbohydrate Counting: A How-to-Teach Guide for Health Professional*, 2nd edition. Alexandria, VA, American Diabetes Association, 2001

Index

Note: Page numbers followed by an *f* refer to figures. Page numbers followed by a *t* refer to tables. Page numbers in **bold** indicate an in-depth discussion.